ORIENTATION AND EVALUATION OF
THE PROFESSIONAL NURSE

ORIENTATION AND EVALUATION OF THE PROFESSIONAL NURSE

MILDRED HILLIARD, R.N., B.S., M.S.

Director of Nursing Service,
St. Louis University Hospitals;
Assistant Professor,
St. Louis University School of Nursing
and Allied Health Services,
St. Louis, Missouri

with 31 *figures*

THE C. V. MOSBY COMPANY

SAINT LOUIS 1974

Printed in the United States of America

Distributed in Great Britain by Henry Kimpton, London

Library of Congress Cataloging in Publication Data

Hilliard, Mildred, 1911-
Orientation and evaluation of the professional nurse.

1. Nurses and nursing. I. Title. [DNLM: 1. Nursing. 2. Patient care team. WY100 H654o 1974]
RT82.H54.H54 610.73'07'15 74-7256
ISBN 0-8016-2190-9

CB/CB/CB 9 8 7 6 5 4 3 2 1

PREFACE

For several years I have been concerned with the mounting cost of inservice orientation programs and with their futility, shown in the results of these programs. The frustration, lack of job satisfaction, and rapid turnover have been with us for a decade, yet little concern with change has been apparent.

Planned change involves the learning of new concepts and ideas, new attitudes and values, and new patterns of behavior and skills. The change agent must realize that staff members are committed to their old habits of behavior and will resist anything that is new or different. If a new approach is planned for orientation, it must be planned in sufficient detail so that the staff members will understand how they get to there from here.

Orientation and Evaluation of the Professional Nurse is based on the philosophy of self-directed learning. It is assumed that young graduates have completed an educational program that has prepared them for participation in the delivery of nursing care to hospitalized patients. The use of self-directed learning techniques and independent study is well established, both in general and in nursing education. To make a smooth transition into practice, the professional nurse needs to observe role models and to have readily available copies of hospital policies, procedure manuals, and reference materials.

Given the proper tools as a guide and the assistance of a clinical nurse when help is needed, the graduate nurse can start practice and make significant contributions to the patient care team. Independent nursing judgments and scientifically based participation in the patient's nursing care plan will improve rapidly through self-directed learning.

I wish to acknowledge my indebtedness to the clinical nurses and other nursing personnel for their support and contributions. I also wish to acknowledge the help extended by Dr. Richard Beeson, Associate Professor in Research Methodology, for his review and suggestions relating to the measurement techniques used. Special thanks go to Joan Carter, Lee Stoll, and Marjorie Koziatek, who helped write the procedures and assisted with the field testing of the program, and to Linda Cross for her many hours of meticulous typing.

Mildred Hilliard

CONTENTS

CHAPTER 1

The problem, determinant, and prescription

PROBLEM

The 1960s were marked by a proliferation of inservice education and orientation programs. The primary goal of the inservice orientation program is to enable the professional nurse to function at her highest level of competence and accountability in the delivery of quality nursing care to the hospitalized patient. Yet, despite the fact that most departments of nursing service in this nation have as one function the provision and implementation of an inservice education program that includes orientation, we still have the same old problem, which has been with us for ten to fifteen years. The problem is twofold:

1. The young professional nurse finds realities in the actual world of hospital nursing so traumatic that she has difficulty in functioning, even after orientation programs that many range from four to twelve weeks in length.
2. The director of nursing and her assistants find it difficult to believe the mistakes the young graduate makes and the insecurity with which she functions.

Origin of orientation programs

It has long been argued by educators in nursing that persons completing their programs would be able to function properly if only the departments of nursing service were properly organized to give nursing care as the students had been taught. They have, further, recommended thorough orientation programs to prepare the young graduate for the nursing role.

Programs to meet these objectives have been brought about by pressure from other groups distinct from the educators. In 1962 the American Hospital Association included, among the functions specified for nursing service departments, the provision and implementation of a program for inservice education. The American Nurses' Association (1964) and the National League for Nursing (1958) have made the same recommendations.

Situation

We take no issue with the use of continuing and inservice education programs, but we believe there is evidence that the orientation programs have not been as effective as they were conceived to be. Some support for the contention that our orientation programs have not been successful was found in a research study (1968 to 1972) by Marlene Kramer, Ph.D., University of California, San Francisco Medical Center, which revealed some shocking facts. This study was concerned with the work adjustment and career patterns of collegiate nurses and with the effect of structural properties and characteristics of the organization on their satisfaction with nursing. Some of the findings of Kramer's research showed that, of the nurses studied, about 20% were in their first job at the end of one year after graduation, about 45% were in their second job, and 15% were in their third job; 20% were in jobs other than hospital nursing. A report of this study, in book form, is being published in 1974.

Nurses—supply and demand

About two thirds of all active professional nurses are employed in hospitals and related institutions. Of this portion, approximately 85% work in short-term general hospitals. Increased use of such hospitals will, therefore, be a major factor in determining future demands for nurses. Projections indicate that growth in the size of the population and changes in its age distribution, together with a continuation of the trend toward greater use of hospitals, will cause hospital patient days to rise by 38% in the 1965-1975 period. Early indications are that Medicare has brought an increase of as much as 15% to 20% in the use of hospitals by persons over 65 years of age; if these indications prove to be correct, this program will add another 4% to hospital use over the longer run, raising the total expected increase to 42%.

If the ratio of professional nurses to patients is assumed to rise by 10% in the next decade, as it did in the last, a 42% growth in hospital patient days should be accompanied by a 56% increase in hospital employment of professional nurses. If the same rates of increase apply to other health institutions, total institutional requirements for nurses will grow by approximately 210,000 between 1965 and 1975. Although demands from other sources (physicians' or dentists' offices, private duty, public health, industrial or occupational health, and nursing education) are expected to grow less quickly, they may still be sufficient to generate demands for approximately 80,000 additional nurses.

These projections indicate a rise of approximately 300,000 in overall *demand* for nurses to a total of 900,000 by 1975. If recent trends in the production and attrition rates of nurses continue, the *supply* of active nurses will increase by about 200,000 to a total of 800,000 by 1975. It thus appears that the growth in demand during this period will exceed growth in supply by about 100,000 nurses, further exaggerating what is already considered by many to be a critical shortage.

In contrast to the situation for physicians and dentists, the present and projected shortages of nurses do not reflect a shortage of training facilities or of nursing graduates. More places are available in nursing schools than there are candidates to fill them. Even more important, between 500,000 and 600,000 qualified nurses are not currently active in the nursing profession, although almost 300,000 of these have kept their licenses and registrations valid.

DETERMINANT

The bifurcation of nursing service and nursing education has gone on for many years. Historically, nursing education and nursing service were once combined in the Diploma School of Nursing. When the education process moved from the hospital to separate institutions, much of the nursing leadership moved to nursing education institutions. The educators did all planning and decision making for the educational process. Many educators, however, actually did not work in the agencies enough to remain expert practitioners.

Not long ago, while an instructor and a student nurse were in a patient's room, the patient suffered a cardiac arrest and the student starting running out of the room. The instructor called to the student to return to the patient. But the student called back over her shoulder, as she continued running: "Nothing doing; I'm going after a nurse who knows what she is doing."

There is no doubt that at that same time the agencies were in need of better-prepared clinical directors.

These conditions have improved markedly over the past few years. Most educators today are competent practitioners, and most clinical directors are well prepared for managing nursing practice and working cooperatively with educators in joint planning for education and clinical practice.

Yet this bifurcation remains and is well documented in the literature. The National Commission for the Study of Nursing and Nursing Education (1970) recommended that

> Nursing leadership work actively to bring education and service together in joint planning and decision making, and that where practicable
> a. Nurse practitioners and clinical directors of nursing service receive significant appointments to (or relevant association with) institutions for nursing education
> b. Nursing faculty in institutions for nursing education be given responsibility for providing or organizing significant elements of nursing care*

The National League for Nursing in its 1973 convention discussed the need for bridging the gap between nursing education and nursing service. As a result an Interdisciplinary Task Force, made up of representatives from the Council of Hospital and Related Institutional Nursing Services, the Council of Home Health Agencies, Community Health Services, and the Council of Baccalaureate and Higher Degree Programs, held its first meeting. The purpose of the meeting was to explore and define dimensions for action to provide quality nursing care through the joint efforts of nursing service and nursing education.

*From National Commission for the Study of Nursing and Nursing Education: An abstract for action, New York, 1970, McGraw-Hill Book Co.

Bifurcation backlash

The young graduate has been the victim of this bifurcation. During her educational program she has heard her instructors complain about the clinical area. She has been told she will find it difficult to practice nursing as she has been taught.

When she arrives in her first job she is given a four- to twelve-week orientation program, partially because the nursing service department feels that the educational institution did not prepare the young graduate to fulfill her job responsibilities.

The young graduate then goes to her assigned area. The nursing staff members, including the L.P.N.s and the nurses' aides, let her know in many ways that she really does not know how to give patient care. By this point in time the young graduate is totally confused, frustrated, and very insecure. No wonder she feels moral outrage and cannot function.

PRESCRIPTION

1. Discontinue the long orientation program.
2. Allow the young graduate to participate, without close supervision, in the delivery of nursing care to hospitalized patients.
3. Let the young graduate utilize self-directed learning and ask for help when she feels she needs it.
4. Give her the respect and support she deserves.
5. Do not criticize her educational program or her instructors.

In line with this prescription, we have introduced a completely new approach to orientation—a program that consists of one week of orientation followed by four weeks of participation in the delivery of nursing care, in which self-directed learning is utilized. Clinical practitioners are available for help and consultation at the request of the young graduate. The sixth week the nurse will be evaluated for competence and accountability.

In May of 1973, when this orientation program was introduced, twenty-five graduates were interviewed for employment. During the interviews the nurses were told that it was our belief that they had received the best possible educational program their school could provide. We would like to test the hypothesis that they could now be given a one-week orientation to the social and organizational structure of the hospital and then be allowed to take their place in the department of nursing, giving and participating in the delivery of nursing care. They were also told that each would be given a manual when she reported for duty and was to return the manual when she finished the six-week experience.

Nurses would be evaluated at the completion of the six-week period, if they did not then attain a score of 80 or higher, they would not be retained as permanent employees.

We had anticipated that this particular part of the discussion would invoke some anxious moments on the part of the new graduates. To our surprise it seemed to create a greater enthusiasm on the part of these nurses. All assured us that they expected to score higher than 80 but that if by chance they did not they believed they would deserve to be terminated.

During the interviews one of the graduates of the Associate Degree Program asked me if I *really* believed she had received an educational program sufficient to allow her to function with the nursing team with competence and accountability. When I assured her that I really did believe she could start participating in the delivery of nursing care if she was willing to use the resources available to her for self-directed learning, her face reflected surprise and delight. Her smile was one of the most spontaneous and sincere I have ever had the pleasure of seeing. She said she had somehow gotten the impression that the Associate Degree Program was a second-rate program.

CHAPTER 2

Process and measurement

FIRST WEEK—Hospital environment

The first week of orientation will be spent in the inservice department. During this week the nurse will be given a short history of the organization. A film tour of all departments will be provided.

The nurse will then be given a set of the department of nursing's standards for nursing care, which will be reviewed thoroughly. The personnel policy manual will be reviewed.

The staffing secretary will discuss tours of duty and special requests for time off. On Friday of the first week the nurse will be given a copy of the orientation manual, which should be returned on Friday of the sixth week.

The nurse is then taken to her assigned area and introduced to all unit personnel.

SECOND WEEK—Unit environment

The professional nurse will be assigned 14 to 18 units (as defined in Chapter 3) of direct patient care as a team member. During this week she should observe the activities of other team members and the team leader.

She will also have the opportunity to assist with any procedures or activities that are not familiar to her.

THIRD WEEK—Skills orientation

The nurse will administer medications and intravenous fluids and have practice in charting and maintaining nursing records. This will give her an opportunity to develop skills in organizing her task-oriented functions and to develop speed in the delivery of care using these technical skills.

FOURTH WEEK—Leadership skills

The nurse will function, under supervision, as a team leader in the area of assignment.

Objectives and behaviors—Team leader

1. *Objective:* To demonstrate knowledge of basic principles of leadership.
   Behavior:
   Demonstrates knowledge of leadership roles and relationships.
   Demonstrates knowledge of the basic concepts of leadership.
   Identifies selected leadership patterns.
   Demonstrates ability to discriminate the proper leadership pattern applicable to a specific situation.
   Identifies selected leadership functions.
   Classifies leadership functions according to desired goals achieved by means of the interim activities.
2. *Objective:* To develop increased understanding of the concepts of human behavior as a basis for understanding of self and others.
   Behavior:
   Utilizes knowledge that the basic needs of man influence behavior.
   Identifies and copes with own feelings in a constructive manner.
   Identifies and constructively directs behavior reflected by feelings.
   Establishes realistic expectations for self.
   Utilizes assets to adjust to her limitations.
   Assists others to express and clarify their ideas and feelings.
   Demonstrates insight into the concept of individual differences.
3. *Objective:* To develop understanding of leadership roles and responsibilities in contemporary nursing practice.
   Behavior:
   Utilizes proper channels of communication within the organizational structure.
   Demonstrates insight into the changing trends of nursing practice and the challenges that are offered for future development.
   Demonstrates positive attitudes toward change and the acceptance and implementation of change in the hospital environment.
   Participates actively in discussions with members of the health team.
   Assumes responsibility for developing team members to upgrade the quality of patient care.
4. *Objective:* To demonstrate skill in planning, coordinating, supervising, and evaluating nursing care for a group of persons.
   Behavior:
   Demonstrates understanding of the team approach concept as a means of providing for proficient patient care.
   Interprets influence of the social and cultural environment on the patient and integrates these concepts in nursing care.
   Interprets needs through the overt behavior of the patient.
   Demonstrates insight in interpreting covert behavior.
   Selects pertinent resources in formulating a nursing care plan.
   Utilizes and interprets importance of family relationships in patient care.
   Analyzes effectiveness of nursing care in relation to the goal.

a. Confers with nursing team in formulating a workable plan of nursing care.
b. Analyzes nursing care plan with the nursing team.
c. Revises plan and goals as necessary to render effective nursing care.
d. Uses nursing care plan as a guide for providing continuity of patient care.

Demonstrates insight concerning application of scientific principles to nursing care.

Records and reports to the appropriate team member pertinent information relating to the patient.

Applies principles of democracy in directing the activities of others.

Performs responsibilities in accord with a hierarchy of values.

Asserts self and demonstrates initiative in self-direction.

Demonstrates kindness and willingness to help others by her words and actions.

Assumes responsibility for her actions.

Demonstrates awareness of the legal implications inherent in her professional practice.

This fourth week of orientation will be under the direction and supervision of the nurse clinician.

FIFTH WEEK—Leadership and managerial skills

During the fifth week the R.N. will function independently but receive any assistance or counseling she requests. The clinical nurse will do two audits with the new R.N. during the week.

SIXTH WEEK—Evaluation of competence and accountability

During the sixth week the R.N. will be evaluated. She will be observed during team conferences, while walking rounds, and in other activities required of the team leader.

The nurse competency rating scale included here was developed to be used in conjunction with the scores from audits utilizing *Standards of Nursing Care: A Guide for Evaluation.* Scores from these two measurement techniques will be used to evaluate the competence of the new graduate nurse at the completion of a six-week orientation and evaluation period.

The nurse competency rating scale has numerical values assigned to each behavior. The final score for each nurse, on the competency rating scale, is the mean score derived from the sum of the total scores for each of the component rating scales. These rating scales were designed to include the specific activities and interactions expected of the team leader.

The use of numerical values rather than a rating scale of A, B, C, etc. was an arbitrary decision. This system was selected to provide consistency with the audit scores, which are numerical.

The scale will be rated by clinical nurse practitioners who are experienced in the giving of patient care and have had experience in teaching in an institution of nursing education. The rating scale will be scored after (preferably) no less than five observations of these various functions during actual performance of the activity being rated.

During the evaluation period in the sixth week five patient audits will be done. Selection of the patients will be at random from the group of patients receiving their nursing care under the direction of the professional nurse being evaluated.

Scoring

The five audits provide for 15 yes scores and 15 total scores. The final score on the patient audits is obtained by dividing the sum of the yes scores by the sum of the total scores.

The competency rating scale combines five observation ratings, representing appropriate numerical values, for each statement on the rating scale. The average of the ratings obtained for a statement under consideration is recorded as the score on that item. When scores on all the items listed under a given area of nursing responsibility have been added and their average determined, the resulting value is the score for that rating area. Six areas of nursing responsibility are included in this scale, and the final score on the competency rating scale will be the average score that is obtained from these six area scores. This rating scale therefore yields an observational appraisal of the overall competence of the professional nurse.

A sample tabulation, showing how the rating scale is used, has been marked for one of the six areas covered (professionalism) and can serve as a scoring guide for each section of the nurse competency rating scale.

The individual nurse will have two final scores. One is the score from the nursing care audits. The audit scores evaluate the quality of the care patients received under the participation and leadership of the nurse who is being evaluated. The second, from the competency rating scale, evaluates the extent to which the nurse is competent and accountable in her interactions.

Evaluation record follows.

Newly appointed professional nurse's evaluation record

Evaluation period ______________________

Name, R.N. ______________________ Rater ______________________

Audit scores

		YES	TOTAL
Audit 1			
	K	12	16
	R	11	14
	E	43	47
Audit 2			
	K	14	15
	R	16	20
	E	44	46
Audit 3			
	K	12	18
	R	16	20
	E	52	56
Audit 4			
	K	18	22
	R	16	20
	E	48	54
Audit 5			
	K	20	24
	R	18	22
	E	50	54
Totals		390	448
Score		.87	

Competency rating scale

AREA OF RATING	SCORE
Professionalism	92.2
Team leader responsibilities	90.4
Assignment sheet	98
Team conference	92.6
Walking-planning rounds	93.5
Change-of-shift report	96
Total average score	93.8

Key:

1	Excellent	100
2	Superior	90
3	Average	80
4	Below average	70
5	Unsatisfactory	60
6	Score	

Legend:

K (Kardex) = Nursing care plan
R = Patient chart record
E = Patient and environment

Key:

$$\frac{\text{Yes } 390}{\text{Total } 448} = \text{Score } .87\ (87\%)$$

FINAL SCORES

Nursing care audits	.87
Competency rating scale	93.8

Nurse competency rating scale

PROFESSIONALISM

	1	2	3	4	5	6
1. Belongs to her professional organization.				√		70
2. Adheres to code of the professional nurse.			√			80
3. Is neat and well groomed. Follows dress code of the organization to which she belongs.	√ √	√	√	√		88
4. Cooperates with unit and hospital regulations.	√ √ √ √ √					100
5. Reports on and off duty promptly.	√ √ √		√ √			92

	1	2	3	4	5	6
6. Takes responsibility for her own learning.	✓✓ ✓✓✓					100
7. Is self-directing: takes initiative and goes ahead on her own.	✓✓ ✓✓ ✓					100
8. Makes decisions willingly and appropriately.	✓		✓✓ ✓✓			84
9. If unsure, consults policy or procedure manual and reference material; if unable to ascertain answers, consults clinical nurse or supervisor.	✓✓ ✓✓ ✓					100
10. Contributes as member of the health team in planning and evaluating patient care.	✓✓ ✓ ✓✓					100
11. Is reliable: keeps healthy and is on duty when assigned; follows through with responsibilities.	✓✓ ✓✓ ✓					100
12. Impresses others with sincerity and concern for patient care.						
13. Participates in staff meetings.						
14. Is considerate and helpful to all unit personnel.						
AREA SCORE						92.2

TEAM LEADER RESPONSIBILITIES

	1	2	3	4	5	6
1. Counts narcotics with nurse from previous shift.						
2. Makes any needed adjustments in assignment sheet.						
3. Listens to change-of-shift report.						
4. Makes rounds with attending physician or resident house staff.						
5. Makes walking rounds with team members for clarification of patient care.						
6. Confers with unit manager on transfers, tests, discharge, or other administrative problems.						
7. Reports to unit manager regarding housekeeping, maintenance, supplies, and equipment.						
8. Plans, directs, and assists with bedside nursing care given to patients on her team.						
9. Makes rounds as frequently as necessary for the purpose of observing, assessing, and meeting patient needs and supervising or assisting personnel for whom she is responsible.						
10. Instructs both the patient and the family of all patients who are going to surgery and completes the preoperative checklist.						
11. Visits all postoperative patients immediately on their return to unit.						

Continued.

Nurse competency rating scale—cont'd

TEAM LEADER RESPONSIBILITIES—cont'd	1	2	3	4	5	6
12. Sees all emergencies immediately; also reports all incidental mishaps to the nursing office and makes out an incident report, one copy only.						
13. Assists physicians as indicated in examination of patients, performing diagnostic tests, changing dressings, etc.						
14. Requests unit manager to call the chaplain, at request of the patient or his family, for any patient going to surgery who is not on the published schedule and for all patients placed on the critical list or deceased.						
15. Spot-checks transcription of doctor's orders for accuracy.						
16. Conducts daily team conference.						
17. Checks team members frequently for performance of duties and quality of care.						
18. Checks team members' charting daily and signs nursing notes when checked.						
19. Makes assignments for the following day by 2:30 P.M.						
20. Checks to see that all team members have finished their daily assignment and charting. Checks environment, including bathrooms.						
21. Tape-records change-of-shift report.						
22. Prepares census and condition sheet.						
23. Prepares nursing report for the nursing office.						
24. Reports any emergencies that would prevent completing the day's assignments, by 2:30 P.M. This would allow sufficient time for float personnel to assist the team in assignment and finishing by 3:30 P.M. (or end of shift).						
25. Counts narcotics with oncoming nurse at 3, 11, or 7 A.M.						
26. Gives an appropriate, taped change-of-shift report.						
27. Reports off duty promptly at 3:30, 11:30, or 7:30 A.M.						

ASSIGNMENT SHEET	1	2	3	4	5	6
1. All nursing personnel are listed by name and position (example: Ms. M. Brown, R.N.)						
2. Assignment sheet indicates the date and shift.						
3. Patients are listed by name and room number.						
4. Break time (not to be before 9:30 A.M.) and lunch hour are designated.						

	1	2	3	4	5	6
5. Time for team conference is designated; the name or topic of the conference is indicated.						
6. Team members responsible for patients while team conference is going on are listed.						
7. Assignment board is kept at the desk in a designated place.						
8. Team member is not assigned more than 14 to 20 units of work except in extreme emergencies.						
9. Functional activities are assigned; assignments for hospital personnel are on white forms; green forms are used for baccalaureate students and pink for board of education students.						

TEAM CONFERENCE	1	2	3	4	5	6
1. Conference time is designated on assignment sheet.						
2. Conference lasts no longer than 20 minutes.						
3. Person assigned to the patient under discussion gives a short report of the care given the patient and lists any observations.						
4. Other team members may give observations and suggestions for care.						
5. Plan of care is outlined, utilizing suggestions from all team members.						
6. Other patients are discussed briefly and any changes or observations noted.						
7. Team leader utilizes all opportunities for teaching.						
8. Asks opinion of all team members during discussion.						
9. Keeps notes so she can update care plans.						
10. Ends conference promptly.						

WALKING-PLANNING ROUNDS	1	2	3	4	5	6
1. Introduces herself and team member who will give care for the shift.						
2. Explains any test, procedures, or the day's routine to the patient.						
3. Maintains focus of conversation with co-workers and patient on matters about the patient and his immediate care.						
4. Speaks clearly and makes sure orders are understood.						
5. Allows members to make suggestions when principles are not compromised.						

Continued.

Nurse competency rating scale—cont'd

WALKING-PLANNING ROUNDS—cont'd	1	2	3	4	5	6
6. Promotes attitude of professionals in all team members during rounds.						
7. Makes team members feel needed and understood.						
8. Addresses patient by name and shows respect.						
9. Accepts expressions of complaint and assures patient she will return to effect any changes necessary.						
10. Comments about patient's actions, to remind and reassure him of signs of improvement.						
11. Does not utilize more than 20 to 30 minutes in walking rounds—14 to 18 patients.						

CHANGE-OF-SHIFT REPORT	1	2	3	4	5	6
1. Date, time, team recorder.						
2. Each patient is identified by status (Mr., Mrs., Miss), name, age, room and bed, diagnosis, and doctor.						
3. Reports only pertinent *new* or *changed* information: a. Condition b. Observations c. Diagnostic test, medications, surgery d. Complications e. Brief medical history f. Basic needs g. Patient or family reactions h. Problems i. Discharge plans						
4. At conclusion gives any general messages that are of importance, such as that surgeons have made rounds or that all 7:30 medications have been given.						

CUES FOR NURSE COMPETENCY RATING SCALE

Professionalism

1. Belongs to her professional organization.
   a. Rating should be 1 if she belongs, since many of the professional nurses do not belong to A.N.A.
   b. If the nurse does not belong, her rating should be 4.
2. Adheres to code of the professional nurse. The code for nurses, adopted by the American Nurses' Association in 1950 and revised in 1960 and 1968, is intended to serve the individual practitioner as a guide to the ethical principles that should govern her nursing practice, conduct, and relationship.

Code

I. The nurse provides services with respect for the dignity of man, unrestricted by consideration of nationality, race, creed, color, or status.
II. The nurse safeguards the individual's right to privacy by judiciously protecting information of a confidential nature, sharing only that information relevant to his care.
III. The nurse maintains individual competence in nursing practice, recognizing and accepting responsibility for individual actions and judgment.
IV. The nurse acts to safeguard the patient when his care and safety are affected by incompetent, unethical, or illegal conduct of any person.
V. The nurse uses individual competence as a criterion in accepting delegated responsibilities and assigning nursing activities to others.
VI. The nurse participates in research activities when assured that the rights of individual subjects are protected.
VII. The nurse participates in the efforts of the profession to define and upgrade standards of nursing practice and education.
VIII. The nurse, acting through the professional organization, participates in establishing and maintaining conditions of employment conducive to high-quality nursing care.
IX. The nurse works with members of the health professions and other citizens in promoting efforts to meet health needs of the public.
X. The nurse refuses to give or imply endorsement to advertising, promotion, or sales for commercial products, service, or enterprises.*

   a. Develops effective care plans on all patients.
   b. Does not divulge sensitive information given her by the patient.
   c. Uses unit's library resources to improve her competencies.
   d. Participates in research projects concerning nursing.
   e. Participates in efforts of the staff in upgrading the standards of nursing care.
   f. Makes rounds with the medical staff and consults social service and other health professionals regarding patient care.

3. Is neat and well groomed.
   a. Follows dress code of the organization.
   b. Hair is short or pinned back.
   c. Shoes and uniform are clean.
   d. Cap is optional.
   e. Uniform length is neither micro, mini, nor maxi; white hose only are worn.
   f. Wears name pin at all times when she is on duty.
4. Cooperates with unit and hospital rules and regulations.
   a. Does not give information concerning patients to the press or to unauthorized persons.
   b. Reports inappropriate behavior taking place on her unit.
   c. Makes out incident reports on all accidents, use of wrong medication or treatment, omission of medication or therapy, or any other incident of major importance.
5. Reports on and off duty promptly.

*Code for nurses with interpretive statements, prepared by the American Nurses' Association, Kansas City, Mo.

   a. Calls to say she will be late if unexpected emergencies occur.
6. Takes responsibility for her own learning.
   a. Uses the unit library and procedure book or policy manual to learn about patient diagnoses, medications, and treatments or about rules and regulations.
7. Is self-directing: takes initiative and goes ahead on her own.
   a. Identifies and performs extra tasks with patients and personnel.
   b. Talks to patients who are discouraged or confused.
   c. Offers comfort such as talking, water, or juice to patients.
   d. Finds time to help and teach ancillary personnel.
   e. Is considerate of relatives and spends time explaining care given the patient.
8. Makes decisions willingly and appropriately.
   a. Knows plan of care and makes adjustments where necessary.
9. If unsure, consults policy or procedure manual or reference material or (if unable to ascertain answer) consults clinical nurse or supervisor.
   a. Asks for help in doubtful situations, to avoid making errors.
   b. Views situation herself, instead of depending on reports alone.
   c. Periodically reviews assignment and work accomplished by herself and team members.
10. Contributes as a member of the health team in planning and evaluating patient care.
   a. Reports observations that would have a bearing on a patient's health care plan.
   b. Makes rounds with the medical staff and collaborates in planning care.
11. Is reliable: keeps healthy and makes every effort to be on duty when assigned.
   a. Takes her yearly medical checkup promptly when requested.
   b. Seeks medical help when she is ill.
   c. Reports situation if work is not completed. Asks for help when she needs help.

Team leader responsibilities

1. Counts narcotics with the nurse from the previous shift.
   a. Narcotics are an important legal responsibility. There is no way to relieve yourself of legal complications unless you count the narcotics when you receive the keys and responsibility.
2. Makes any needed adjustments in assignment sheet.
   a. Makes adjustments in assignment sheet to reflect any changes on the midnight census sheet.
   b. Hangs assignment sheet in the proper designated spot.
   c. Team members should know their assignments by 10 minutes after the hour. This should make it unnecessary for the team leader to carry the assignment board with her.
3. Listens to change-of-shift report.

a. Listens to report of the entire hall.
b. Makes notes of changes in medical or nursing care plan.
c. Makes notes of communications that need clarification before the team leader of the previous shift leaves.
d. Makes notes of events needing her immediate attention.

4. Makes rounds with attending physician or resident house staff.
   a. Takes Kardex and scratch pad with her.
   b. Is alert and stands close enough to the chief resident or the private physician to communicate regarding patient observations or needs.
   c. Is quiet and attentive; does not indulge in conversation with others accompanying the rounds.
   d. Turns off (or down) loud radio or TV that may be interfering with communications.
5. Makes walking rounds with team members for clarification of patient care assignments.
   a. Includes patient in the discussion; introduces both herself, if not known, and the person who will give care during the shift.
   b. Speaks clearly enough to be understood by team members.
   c. Does not spend undue time while in clarification rounds. Tells patient she will return for discussions needing more time.
   d. Limits her walking rounds to no more than 20 minutes.
6. Confers with unit manager on transfers, discharges, admissions, tests, and other administrative activities.
   a. Ascertains her discharges for the day and plans time for last-minute instructions.
   b. Makes sure that transporter, someone from patient services, or a member of the nursing staff accompanies the patient to the correct street exit and assists him in getting into his mode of transportation.
   c. Consults unit manager about equipment that is required and not available.
   d. Consults nursing office about equipment requests from outside vendors. (Anything not coming from the storeroom or Central Service.)
   e. Reports, to nursing office, all patient elopements or patients leaving without medical consent.
7. Reports to unit manager regarding housekeeping, maintenance, supplies, and equipment.
   a. Does not use valuable time looking for equipment; requests it from the unit manager.
   b. Reminds unit manager of dirty bathrooms, torn curtains, etc.
8. Plans, directs, and assists with bedside nursing care given to patients in her assigned area.
   a. Checks with her team members frequently enough to know what they are doing and supervises where needed.
   b. Uses every opportunity to do incidental teaching.
   c. Makes sure her team members know the plan of care.

9. Makes rounds as frequently as necessary for the purposes of observing, assessing, and meeting patient needs and supervising or assisting personnel for whom she is responsible.
   a. Makes rounds frequently to observe patients.
   b. Keeps physician informed of drastic changes in patient conditions.
10. Instructs patient and the family of each patient going to surgery and completes the preoperative checklist.
    a. After operative schedule arrives on the hall, about 2:30 P.M., checks to see that unit secretary attaches a checklist to the front of the chart and starts the checklist.
    b. Talks to patient, to make sure he knows he is going to surgery.
    c. Talks to family, to clarify any questions relating to surgery.
11. Visits all postoperative patients immediately on their return to unit.
    a. Visits, checks condition, and makes note on the nurses' progress record.
    b. Notifies physician of any problem relating to recovery.
12. Sees all emergencies immediately. Reports all incidental mishaps or injuries to the nursing office and makes out an incident report when indicated. (Incident reports are made in one copy only.)
    a. Checks immediately, after all emergency admissions, to assess requirement for equipment, supplies, and personnel to care for the patient.
    b. Sees relatives immediately on their arrival, to reassure or give any information that can be given at the time.
    c. Protects clothing or valuables. These are placed under the bed until the unit manager can arrive and take charge of belongings.
13. Assists physicians as indicated in examination of patients, performing diagnostic tests, changing dressings, etc.
    a. Has responsibility to assist physician and medical students during physical examination of all female patients.
    b. Procedures and diagnostic tests require two persons, in many cases, for technique to remain free of contamination.
    c. Must be ever conscious of hand washing, before and after each procedure.
14. Requests unit manager to call the chaplain at request of the patient or his family, for patients going to surgery, who are not on the published schedule, and for all patients placed on the critical list or deceased.
    a. Chaplain is called for all the patients just specified, regardless of whether they are Catholic or not.
15. Spot-checks transcription of doctor's orders for accuracy.
    a. If nurse is in doubt about a transcribed order, she should check the doctor's order sheet.
    b. Spot-checks occasionally for accuracy and for A.M. or P.M. notation.
16. Conducts daily team conference.
    a. Sees that conference is properly scheduled on the assignment sheet.
    b. Time, place, and topic should be noted.
17. Checks team members frequently for performance of duties and quality of care.

18. Checks team members' charting daily and signs notes when she checks.
19. Makes assignments for the following day by 2:30 P.M.
    a. Next day's assignments are then placed on the assignment clipboard underneath the list of current day's assignments.
20. Checks to see that all team members have finished their daily assignments and charting.
    a. Team members should not all be charting at the same time; this activity should be staggered so that some team members are free to answer lights.
    b. If team members are behind in their work, makes adjustments so that all members can be off duty on time.
    c. Sees that rooms and environment are clean and in order before change of shift.
21. No cues.
22. Prepares census and condition sheet.
    a. Is as accurate as possible in assessing points.
    b. Makes sure that condition of each patient is recorded.
23. Prepares nursing report for the nursing office.
    a. Nursing report should list all critical patients, all VIPs, and anything else that should be brought to the attention of the office, such as accidents or changes in condition.
24. Reports any emergencies that would prevent completion of the day's assignment, by 2:30 P.M. This will allow sufficient time for float personnel to assist in care.
    a. Assesses progress of work.
    b. Is mindful of time at all times so that care can be given in a reasonable length of time.
25. Counts narcotics with oncoming nurse.
    a. Counts and turns over keys to successor.

Assignment sheet—Necessary cues

A. Assignment sheets must be kept in one designated spot at all times.
B. Total units of work should be designated for all assigned team members.
C. No more than 14 to 20 units of work should be assigned to any one person.

Team conference—Necessary cues

A. Leader starts and stops conference on time.
B. Encourages all to participate in discussion.
C. Keeps notes so she can update care plan.
D. Gives summary of discussion at end of time scheduled for conference.

Walking-planning rounds—Necessary cues

A. Team leader introduces herself and the team member who is to give care.
B. All team members are alert and maintain focus of conversation on matters concerning care.
C. No laughing or talking among team members occurs.

D. Team members may make suggestions.
E. Rounds are conducted in a professional manner, with no relaxed, play conduct.
F. Leader speaks clearly and makes sure that instructions are understood.

Change-of-shift report—Necessary cues

A. Includes in taped report the date, time that report was recorded, and name of person recording.
B. Keeps report short but includes all observations and changes in patient status. New and changed items are recorded on the patient Kardex and should be discussed in detail on walking-planning rounds.
C. Records any general messages that should be passed on to the next shift.

The nursing audit*

THE PATIENT AND HIS ENVIRONMENT

General nursing care measures for hospitalized patients

GROUP I: Nursing interventions that are necessary to maintain hygiene, physical comfort, activity, body mechanics, rest and sleep, and safety

A. Hygiene and physical comfort
   1. Bath, complete or with assistance, as necessary for all patients who
      a. Need it for cleanliness
      b. Need circulatory or skin stimulation
      c. Request or desire bathing
      d. Are inpatients (all patients should be offered the opportunity of daily bathing unless this is contraindicated; for example, no bath is to be given to patients who have had pericardial pain within 2 to 24 hours, until the pain has been adequately assessed)
   2. Opportunities for hand washing will be provided
      a. Before and after each meal
      b. After use of the bedpan or the urinal
   3. Mouth care for patients will consist of
      a. Hygiene measures (brushing, mouthwash, or denture care) at least three times daily after meals
      b. Measures that are noted on Kardex if more frequent care is needed
      c. Denture cup at bedside for patient with dentures
   4. Hair grooming care includes
      a. Daily combing or brushing
      b. Giving special care such as shampoos as needed
      c. Informing patient if barber or beautician is available
      d. Providing stockinette cap or securing a wig for the patient with shaved head
   5. Both fingernails and toenails of the patient will be

*This material (pp. 20 to 41) from Carter, Joan, Hilliard, Mildred, Castles, Mary, Stoll, Lee, and Cowan, Anne: Standards of nursing care: a guide for evaluation, New York, 1972, Springer Publishing Co., Inc.

a. Cleaned
b. Trimmed if indicated (and if not contraindicated)

6. Skin care will consist of
   a. Application of lotion for dryness
   b. Special attention to areas susceptible to breakdown (for example, use of heel protectors, elbow protectors, flotation pads; pressure areas rubbed every 2 hours; patient turned every 2 hours)
   c. Appropriate decubitus care as indicated
   d. Backrub to be offered to every patient every morning with the bath and each evening
   e. Removal of electrodes for cleansing skin every 8 hours if metal electrodes are used or according to the manufacturer's specifications if other types are used
7. Care of patients with dressings, compresses, bandages, binders, elastic stockings, or bandages includes
   a. Removing dressing on transvenous pacemakers and on intracatheters once a day and inspecting the site for evidence of inflammation or infection; if no evidence of phlebitis is noted, a clean dressing is applied, using specified ointment or solution; label the dressing with date, time, type of insertion, and initials
   b. Sending specimen of drainage to the laboratory for culture and sensitivity tests if signs of inflammation or infection are noted at insertion sites and informing the attending physician
   c. Checking other dressings for cleanliness and dryness
   d. Changing dressings when indicated, noting skin irritation
   e. Removing elastic stockings or bandages twice a day for 30 minutes
8. Bed linen should be
   a. Clean, dry, and in good order
   b. Changed daily
9. Special measures for the incapacitated patient who has physical rehabilitation potential include
   a. Teaching adaptation of bath procedure
   b. Assisting patient to use assistive devices appropriately (for example, universal holder for the bath brush, toothbrush, hairbrush)
   c. Teaching adaptation in procedure of getting dressed
   d. Teaching selected patients the rationale of avoiding as much isometric exercise as possible
   e. Observing threshold of fatigue and excessive anxiety; teach the patient within the limits of these realities
   f. Informing patient of community resources

B. Activity and body mechanics
   1. Ambulation of the patient will be carried out
      a. According to physician's directives
      b. According to patient's needs

c. By using proper transfer techniques
d. By assisting with use of adaptive equipment such as crutches, wheelchairs, walkers, lifts, braces, canes

2. Assistance in turning in bed will be given to patients who cannot turn themselves and who need this type of movement
3. Passive or active exercises of extremities (provided condition indicates or permits) are used every 2 hours for patients who
   a. Are confined to bed
   b. Need circulatory stimulation
   c. Need musculoskeletal activity
4. Provision should be made for proper body alignment for the patient by
   a. Appropriate use of traction equipment
   b. Using sandbags, footboards, supports
   c. Using splints, corsets, slings
5. Proper use of turning frames (Stryker frame, CircOlectric bed) includes
   a. Following instructions provided with the equipment
   b. Using safety belts, bolts, and locks provided

C. Rest and sleep
   1. Physical environment should at all times
      a. Be quiet
      b. Have controlled lighting
      c. Have proper ventilation and temperature
   2. Patient can be aided by
      a. Comfortable position
      b. Soothing backrubs
      c. Medication as needed or as order is obtained
      d. Nourishment
      e. Consideration of his usual sleep habits
      f. Adequate rest periods between therapy sessions

D. Safety
   1. For patient safety during ambulation, nursing personnel should
      a. Accompany all patients for their initial ambulation after surgery or after prolonged bed rest
      b. Accompanying patients at other times as necessary
   2. For patient safety during transportation, nursing personnel should
      a. Lock wheels of stretchers, wheelchairs, and beds when a patient is lifted out of or assisted onto them
      b. Use safety belts on all patients who are on stretchers
      c. Secure intravenous poles at the foot end of the stretcher
      d. Pull, rather than push, wheelchair into and out of elevator
      e. Accompany selected patients who must be detached from cardiac monitors or who have intravenous fluids or oxygen therapy to other hospital areas
   3. Bed precautions for patient safety include having

   a. Height of bed low unless personnel are present or safety measures are used
   b. Side rails up, on beds of all patients who
      (1) Are unconscious, confused, delirious
      (2) Have seizures or history of seizures
      (3) Have both eyes covered
      (4) Are recovering from a general anesthetic
      (5) Have received large amounts of sedatives or narcotics
      (6) Are over age 70 (hospital policy)
   c. Call light, tissues, and drinking water within easy reach of patient
4. Restraints are used to prevent patient from harming himself, harming others, or to facilitate treatment only if they are
   a. Ordered by physician or on, pending order by physician (hospital policy)
   b. Properly applied to ensure comfort as well as safety
   c. Properly maintained
5. Environment should be
   a. Mechanically safe—have dry floors, furniture in good repair, and proper placement of machines and equipment
   b. Clean
   c. Free from clutter
   d. Properly lighted
6. Isolation technique should be carried out as set forth by the hospital policy
7. Disposal of wastes should be as follows
   a. Containers for urine, feces, or vomitus are to be emptied immediately unless there is reason to save a specimen for analysis
   b. Dressings must be disposed of properly
8. Special safety precautions should be noted on the individual nursing care plan of any patient who is blind, hard-of-hearing, etc. For example, a patient who has impaired vision should be given a thorough explanation of the kinds and location of foods on the tray.
9. Signs for safety that must be posted on the door or bed are
   a. *No smoking* for oxygen therapy
   b. *Radioactive precautions* for patients with implants
   c. *Isolation* for patients requiring isolation technique
   d. *Blind, hard-of-hearing,* etc., for patients with sensory defects
10. Identification includes
    a. Patient in assigned room and bed
    b. Correct and legible armbands on all patients
11. Equipment regulations include
    a. All equipment should be in proper working order and be checked at least once a day
    b. Supplies should be readily available
    c. Must be placed so that if it falls it will not injure the patient

12. For patient and personnel safety when using electrical equipment, nursing personnel should
    a. Use equipment with 3-prong plugs (no adaptors and no extension cords)
    b. Use only battery-powered razors or radios for patients who are being monitored
    c. Be certain that the external parts of equipment used internally (pacing wires, central venous pressure tubing, intravenous lines) are adequate
    d. Keep all electrical equipment at least 6 inches from the patient's bed
    e. Avoid placing saline bottles or other fluids on electrical equipment
    f. Disconnect cord from the electrical outlet if liquid is spilled on the equipment, wipe dry, and have equipment checked by the maintenance person if there is a question of liquid being on terminals or inner mechanism
    g. Keep environment, including the patient's bed, clean and dry at all times
    h. Avoid overloading electrical outlets
    i. Avoid standing on a wet floor when plugging in or operating electrical equipment
    j. Operate electrical equipment only when hands are dry
    k. Avoid touching a good ground when using the other hand to operate electrical equipment
13. Labels should be affixed to
    a. Bedside medications
    b. Drainage bottles if not clearly identified by location
    c. Drainage tubes if multiple and if not clearly identified by location
    d. Intravenous bottles (giving date, rate, added medication, and signature of the nurse who prepared the solution)
    e. Any intravenous device (indicating what it is, length, size, and date of insertion)
    f. Any monitor that displays the output of transducers sensing intracardiac, blood, or pulmonary pressures

GROUP II: Nursing interventions necessary to maintain oxygen supply, nutrition, elimination, fluid and electrolyte balance, regulatory mechanisms, and sensory functions (Interventions listed in this group imply that the nurse recognizes the body's responses to disease.)

E. Nutrition—fluid and electrolyte balance
   1. Assure proper intake by
      a. Giving oral fluids, intravenous fluids, and tube feedings as indicated
      b. Withholding fluids when necessary
      c. Maintaining adequate food intake
      d. Adjusting consistency of the food
   2. Assess electrolyte status by observing the patient and by reading the laboratory reports

3. Assure proper intravenous therapy by
   a. Following pharmaceutical directives for admixture of intravenous solutions
   b. Applying appropriate stabilizing device
   c. Titrating according to
      (1) Patient's condition
      (2) Objective of therapy
      (3) Strength and kind of solution
   d. Changing site of needle insertion for patients with continuous intravenous therapy at least every 72 hours unless contraindicated
   e. Changing tubing for continuous intravenous therapy once each 24 hours
   f. Checking system for patency or extravasation of fluid into tissue every 30 to 60 minutes, depending on the condition of the patient and the system

F. Elimination
1. Adequacy of bowel elimination should be assessed and maintained by
   a. Checking and recording bowel movements daily
   b. Giving enemas, laxatives, stool softeners, and suppositories when ordered and indicated
   c. Encouraging fluids and activity
   d. Providing bedside commode
2. Adequacy of urine elimination should be assessed and maintained by
   a. Initiating input and output (I & O) records and tests for specific gravity or glucose content on any patient whose condition indicates the need
   b. Observation and recording of voiding—amount and frequency—and amount of bladder distention
   c. Catheterization of patient as indicated
   d. Checking patency and position of catheter, tubing, and drainage container
   e. Using proper irrigating technique
3. Initiation or continuation of bladder-training program as indicated
4. Initiation or continuation of bowel-training program as indicated
5. Provision of perineal care twice daily for patients with indwelling catheters
6. Care of other drainage equipment includes
   a. Checking patency and position of tubes
   b. Irrigating tubes as needed or ordered
   c. Using aseptic technique when handling drainage equipment
   d. Ostomy bag—applying, cleaning, and changing as needed
7. Assessment of drainage includes
   a. Measuring and recording all output
   b. Noting and recording color and consistency of drainage

G. Oxygen and ventilation
1. Measures for providing adequate oxygen and ventilation are

a. Encouraging patient to cough, turn, and deep breathe
   (1) Every 2 hours, unless contraindicated, for
      (a) Immobile bed patients
      (b) Selected medical patients
      (c) Postoperative patients
b. Checking patency and position of tracheostomy tube, endotracheal tube, nasal catheter, cannula, or mask
c. Checking indicator of oxygen flow
d. Using proper technique and equipment for suctioning
e. Keeping tracheostomy site clean
f. Checking respirators for proper functioning
g. Removing ashtrays and electric signal cord from the patient's room when oxygen tent is in use

H. Sensory
   1. Measures to maintain adequate sensory perception include
      a. Proper care of protheses (eyeglasses, hearing aids)
      b. Initiation of frequent verbal interaction with the patient
      c. Audiovisual stimulation for selected patients
      d. Providing reading materials or other diversional activities
      e. Having clock or calendar within the patient's view

I. Physiological responses
   1. Observe and intervene as necessary
      a. Appearance
      b. Vital signs
      c. Level of consciousness
      d. Verbal behavior

J. Other bedside therapy
   1. Provisions should be made to ensure safe and proper therapeutic use of hypothermia, hyperthermia, intravenous flow rate, decubitus care devices, rotation of tourniquets, monitoring devices, peritoneal dialysis, bedside medications, chest drainage bottles, by
      a. Correctly manipulating machines
      b. Providing adequate instructions

GROUP III: Nursing interventions that support the patient and family through their emotional reactions to the patient's illness

K. Meeting emotional needs
   1. Indicate to each patient that he is a respected person by
      a. Considering compatibility of roommate in assigning rooms
      b. Allowing him to wear his own clothes and guarding valuable personal items by use of hospital safe or personal lockers
      c. Encouraging questions from him and his family
      d. Attempting to adjust hospital schedules for the convenience of him and his family
      e. Informing his family about the patient's condition

f. Observing the patient's understanding of and his reaction to physical disability and adjusting nursing behaviors accordingly
g. Staying with him during selected tests or procedures carried out on the nursing unit
h. Taking him to the telephone if necessary and if not contraindicated

2. Listen attentively
3. Observe for and report unusual behavior
4. Encourage members of his family in their support of the patient by making the family welcome
   a. Telephone relatives if indicated
   b. Encourage relatives to visit at mealtime and feed patient if desired
   c. Allow relatives to remain with patient if he desires it and it is appropriate to his condition

L. Considering spiritual needs
1. Nurses should assist the patient by
   a. Informing patient of the religious services available
   b. Obtaining such services if requested or indicated
   c. Providing for privacy
   d. Observing protocols of the patient's religion in such things as diet or ritual

GROUP IV: Nursing interventions that will assist the patient and his family to cope with the illness and necessary life adjustment

M. Information and support for the patient and his family
1. Nurses should assist the patient and family by
   a. Orienting him and his family to the hospital and the room environment on admission—will include giving information about use of the communication systems, mealtimes, and location of toilet facilities
   b. Explaining tests and procedures
   c. Developing care plan with the patient
   d. Obtaining assistance of other health disciplines as necessary
   e. Evaluating effectiveness of teaching, through communication with the patient or his family and through communication with other members of the health team
2. Nurses should prepare both the patient and his family for home care by
   a. Learning details of the life situation to which the patient will return, so that she can teach in keeping with these realities
   b. Promoting self-care as soon as possible
   c. Initiating plans for referral if needed
   d. Working with other members of the health team for discharge planning
   e. Including family members in discharge planning
   f. Counseling patient's family concerning the realities of the patient's rehabilitation

3. If patient is dying, the nurse should
    a. Notify both the family and the physician
    b. Treat family with compassion
    c. Continue to treat the patient with respect
    d. Facilitate religious rites
4. If patient dies, the nurse should
    a. Care for the body in accordance with hospital procedures
    b. Accompany relatives to their car or at least to the hospital exit doors
    c. Transfer patient's body to the morgue in accordance with hospital procedures

Medical-surgical clinical standards
Nursing care index—the patient and his environment

Unit 10-S Date 11/20/73 Time 2 P.M.

Patient audit no. 1 Patient classification 3

Initials of member of committee D. W.

	YES	NO	COMMENT
A. Hygiene and physical comfort			
1. Has patient been bathed and been given skin care as required?	✓		
2. Is patient's mouth clean?	✓		
3. Is patient well grooomed (hair, nails, etc.)?	✓		
4. Has special attention been given to pressure or irritated areas?	✓		
5. Has patient been offered backrubs each A.M. and P.M.?		✓	*Not offered on p.m. shift*
6. Are dressings clean and dry?	✓		
7. Are dressings around puncture sites changed once each day and ointment applied?			
8. Is patient's bed clean, dry, and in good order?	✓		
9. Is independence in activities of daily living supported for the physically incapacitated person?			
B. Activity and body mechanics			
1. Has patient activity (dangling, sitting up in chair, ambulating) been executed as indicated?	✓		
2. Have exercises been given if indicated?			

	YES	NO	COMMENT
3. Has patient been turned as indicated?	✓		
4. Is patient in the position conducive to recovery or to proper therapy?	✓		
5. Are supports (footboards, sandbags, pillows) instituted and used correctly?			
6. Are elastic stockings and bandages properly applied and maintained?			
7. Are splints, corsets, slings applied correctly?			
8. Are turning frames used correctly?			
9. Does patient understand the reason for activity, etc.?	✓		
C. Rest and sleep			
1. Is quiet maintained at night and during rest periods?		✓	*Very noisy at night*
2. Is lighting controlled at all times?	✓		
3. Are room temperature and ventilation adequate and comfortable for patient?		✓	*Too warm*
4. Have comfort measures (repositioning, listening) been used to induce sleep or rest?			
5. Has sleeping medication been offered?			
6. Have rest periods been provided between therapy sessions?	✓		
D. Safety			
1. Has patient been accompanied during his initial activity after bed rest?	✓		
2. Is height of bed adjusted properly?	✓		
3. If side rails are necessary, are they up and in safe working order?			
4. Are restraints used as needed and applied properly?			
5. Are safety precautions used for patients while in chairs or wheelchairs?			
6. Are floors dry and safe?	✓		
7. Is isolation room set up properly?			

Continued.

Medical-surgical clinical standards—cont'd
Nursing care index—the patient and his environment—cont'd

	YES	NO	COMMENT
8. Does patient and/or his family understand the proper isolation technique and the reasons for it?			
9. Are contaminated articles (dressings, bedpans, urinals, etc.) disposed of properly?	√		
10. Is furniture appropriate and safe?	√		
11. Are proper signs displayed for patient safety (no smoking, blind, deaf, n.p.o., etc.)?			
12. Is room uncluttered (by newspapers, drinking cups, etc.)?	√		
13. Is patient in the right room and bed and wearing legible ID band?	√		
14. Are call light and other necessary items (tissues, wastebasket, etc.) within easy reach of patient?	√		
15. Are machines or electrical equipment at bedside properly connected and maintained?			
16. Are precautionary measures used, such as labeling of bedside medications and labeling drainage bottles?			
E. Nutrition—fluid and electrolyte balance			
1. Are oral fluids given, restricted, and recorded as indicated?	√		
2. Are patient's preferences of fluid considered?	√		
3. Are fluids and food within patient's reach?	√		
4. Is fresh drinking water obtained every 8 hours?	√		
5. Is correct bottle of IV fluids, with precise labeling, being administered?			
6. Are IV fluids administered at the proper rate?			
7. Has patient been assisted adequately and promptly with eating?	√		
8. Is there evidence that the patient is receiving the correct diet, or are measures taken to obtain a change?	√		
9. Do both the patient and his family understand the reasons for the special diet, fluid restrictions, etc.?			
10. Is there evidence that measures were taken to instruct the patient and his family on diet?			
F. Elimination			
1. Have measures been instituted for the maintenance of proper bowel function?	√		

	YES	NO	COMMENT
2. Has urinary elimination been properly checked and recorded?		√	*Recorded BR × 3*
3. Has bowel and bladder training been initiated or continued?			
4. Has perineal care been given at least twice daily to patients with catheters?			
5. Are drainage tubes patent and properly connected and positioned?			
6. Are irrigation trays properly maintained (clean, labeled, covered)?			
7. Are ostomy bags properly applied, cleaned, and changed as needed?			
8. Does patient understand his plan for elimination care?			
G. Oxygen and ventilation			
1. Has patient been encouraged to turn, cough, and deep breathe at designated intervals?	√		
2. Is oxygen therapy properly given (rate, humidity, position of catheter)?			
3. Is suction equipment properly set up (clean articles, completeness)?			
4. Is there evidence that oral-nasal suctioning has been done?			
5. Is tracheostomy patent, and the site clean?			
6. Are obturator and a complete new tracheostomy set evident at the bedside?			
7. Are respirators used correctly?			
8. Do both the patient and his family understand the reasons for and the precautions to be used in respiratory therapy?			
H. Sensory			
1. Are eyeglasses, hearing aids, dentures, etc. properly cared for?	√		
2. Are appropriate measures used for effective communication?	√		
3. Are measures such as radio, TV, raised window shades suggested or used to stimulate the nonactive patient?			
4. Has the person with impaired vision been assisted with his mail, phone calls, or other reading material?			

Continued.

Medical-surgical clinical standards—cont'd
Nursing care index—the patient and his environment—cont'd

	YES	NO	COMMENT
I. Physiological responses			
Observe patient's appearance, vital signs, level of consciousness, and behavior; compare coder observations with staff observations to verify the nursing unit record.			
J. Other bedside therapy			
1. Is therapeutic equipment properly applied to the patient?			
2. Has IV tubing been changed at least every 24 hours?			
3. Are instructions for the use of the equipment present and legible?			
K. Meeting emotional needs			
These items are checked in terms of the perception of the situation by the patient or his family. Some of the items refer to information needed by the patient and his family; others refer to supportive nursing technique.			
1. Is patient treated with kindness?	√		
2. Are patient and his roommate compatible (in age and condition), or have measures been instituted to provide for this?	√		
3. Has patient been oriented to the hospital and been informed of mealtimes, communication systems, toilet facilities?	√		
4. Is there evidence that the nurses listen to the patient, encourage questions, and generally make the patient feel at ease?	√		
5. Is there any indication that a nurse stayed with an anxious patient, a fearful patient, a very ill patient?			
6. Is patient wearing his own clothing if he wishes to do so?	√		
7. Are patient's valuables and clothing protected?	√		
8. Does patient's family feel relatively at ease in the hospital setting and free to ask questions?	√		
9. Are adjustments made in the hospital schedules as necessary to accommodate the family?	√		
10. Is family encouraged to be with the patient at mealtime and to assist with feeding occasionally?			
11. Is there evidence that the nurses telephoned the patient's family and/or friends as indicated (request of patient, serious condition, dying patient)?			
12. Are both the dying patient and his family (friends) treated with compassion?			

	YES	NO	COMMENT
L. Considering spiritual needs			
1. Is patient aware of the availability of religious counsel and services?	√		
2. Has priest, minister, or rabbi been informed if patient's condition is critical?			
3. Is protocol of the patient's religion observed by the staff?		√	*No evidence*
M. Patient and family teaching			
1. Has patient teaching been initiated?			
2. Has family been involved in the teaching as necessary?	√		
3. Have persons from other disciplines been utilized as indicated?			
4. Is there evidence that the teaching is progressive and effective?	√		
N. Discharge			
1. Have proper plans for rehabilitation been initiated?			
2. Does patient who is preparing to go home understand plan for his progressive activity and return to wellness?	√		
3. Are referrals made for home care?			
4. Are other services of community agencies obtained?			
5. Are family members included in the discharge planning?	√		
6. Are members of the health team included in the discharge planning?			

Safe care question

In unanimous opinion of the coders, is the nursing care given to this patient unsafe? ____________________

Number of *yes* answers 43

Number of *no* answers 5

Total answered 48

COMMENTS: For an unsafe care vote, explain specifically the reason.

____

____

____

____

____

STANDARDS FOR THE NURSING CARE PLAN (KARDEX)

Requirements for planning individualized patient care should be clearly written on the nursing care plan and placed correctly in the Kardex file.

A. The *profile section* should be accurately completed as to
  1. Admission date and time
  2. Height, weight
  3. Blood pressure on admission
  4. Age
  5. Religion
  6. Fully attended (space for priest or minister to complete)
  7. O.R. procedure, date
  8. Room number
  9. Name
  10. Physician's current diagnosis
  11. Service
  12. Physician
  13. Resident
  14. Intern

B. The *drug section* should be accurately completed as to
  1. Name
  2. Dose
  3. Route of administration
  4. Times per day
  5. Hours
  6. Date started
  7. Date to be discontinued (for narcotics and drugs with specified time limits)
  8. Allergies (in red)

C. Record in the *tests and procedures section* should be accurately completed as to
  1. Dates ordered
  2. Dates scheduled (or date ordered with note if unable to schedule)
  3. Names of tests or procedures

D. The *consultation section* should include
  1. Date
  2. Name of person or type of consultation requested

E. The *daily or serial specimens or tests section* should be completed accurately as to
  1. Date ordered
  2. Name of specimen
  3. Dates, time, and/or frequency of specimen collection

F. The *nursing care section* should be completed accurately as to
  1. Dates
  2. Diet, extra nourishment
  3. Fluid, intake and output
  4. Bath

5. Use of Foley catheter
6. Activity
7. Positioning
8. Special skin care
9. Special mouth care
10. Weight
11. Respiratory aids
12. T.P.R., vital signs
13. Physical therapy, x-ray therapy, other therapy
14. Telephone numbers
15. Disposition of preadmission drugs

The sections on *diet, feed, bath,* and *activity* must be filled in for all patients. Other areas may be left blank if not pertinent to care.

G. The *special needs with plan of care section* should be completed as follows
   1. Observations
   2. Clearly stated goals
   3. Clearly stated interventions
   4. Continuing and current assessment
   5. Reviewed, redated, and initialed at least weekly

H. The *treatment section* (which may be used to note physician's directives even though these are not precisely defined as treatments) should indicate accurately
   1. Date ordered
   2. Type of treatment
   3. Frequency and duration of treatment
   4. Materials to be used

I. Date of last bowel movement

J. The *parenteral fluid section* should accurately indicate
   1. Amount and kind of fluid
   2. Additives
   3. Time span
   4. Date
   5. Time started and time discontinued
   6. Amount remaining at shift change

Nursing care index follows.

Nursing care index—nursing care plan (Kardex)

Unit 10-S Date 11/20/73 Time 2 P.M.

Patient audit no. 1 Patient classification 3

Initials of member of committee D. W.

DEFINITION: Each item must be considered in relation to presence, relevance, and accuracy. Accurate or complete is here interpreted to mean that the information is correct, comprehensive, and written as indicated by the Nursing Care Plan Standards and the hospital procedure for nursing care plans.

	YES	NO	COMMENT
A. Profile section			
1. Is the information filled in accurately?	√		
B. Drug section			
1. Are names of the drugs, doses, routes, times, hours, and dates started accurately stated?	√		
2. If drugs are discontinued, is it noted; and are "discontinued" dates indicated for narcotics and drugs with specified time limits?	√		
3. Are allergies noted accurately?	√		
C. Tests and procedures section			
1. Are dates ordered and dates scheduled filled in; is the completion of the tests indicated?			
2. Are tests or procedures clearly and accurately written?			
D. Consultation section			
1. Is the date of the request indicated; if the test is completed, is it noted?			
2. Is the person to be consulted or the type of consultation noted?			
E. Daily or serial specimens or tests section			
1. Are the dates ordered indicated; if the test is completed, is it noted?			
2. Are the names of specimens clearly written?			
3. Are the dates, times, and/or frequency of serial specimens indicated?			
F. Nursing care section			
1. Are the starting dates indicated for each measure; if necessary for follow-up of nursing care, are discontinued dates noted?	√		

	YES	NO	COMMENT
2. Are the spaces indicating diet, ability to feed self, bath, and activity completed?	√		
3. Are the T.P.R. vital signs, and bowel data spaces completed accurately?	√		
4. Are other spaces pertinent to care accurate?	√		
G. General nursing needs section			
1. Is the plan of care dated or redated (at least weekly) and initialed?		√	*No dates*
2. Are observations stated?		√	
3. Are goals clearly stated and pertinent?		√	
4. Are interventions clearly stated and pertinent?		√	
5. Are observations, goals, and interventions complete?			
H. Treatment and/or special order section			
1. Are treatments and special orders dated; if the treatment is discontinued, is it noted?	√		
2. Are types of treatments and/or special orders indicated with the explicit materials to be used?	√		
3. Are frequencies and durations of treatments indicated?	√		
4. Are the treatments complete?	√		
I. Parenteral fluid section			
1. Are the amounts, kinds, sequence of bottles, and additives accurately stated?			
2. Is the time span and/or rate accurately stated, with the amount remaining at shift change?			
3. Are the dates, patient identification, the times started and the fact of completion indicated?			

Patient census __20__

Number of no. 5 and no. 4 patients on unit __4__

Number of R.N.s assigned to floor __6__

Number of L.P.N.s assigned to floor __5__

Number of aides assigned to floor __4__

Team leader __P. Adams, R.N.__

Person assigned to this patient's care today __M. Cross, L.P.N.__

Number of *yes* answers __12__

Number of *no* answers __4__

Total answered __16__

STANDARDS FOR THE NURSING RECORD (CHART)

Nursing requirements for pertinent communications and record keeping

A. General requirements are
   1. Patient's name and room number on chart folder
   2. Patient's name and room number on all nursing chart forms
   3. Allergy labels on front of chart

B. T.P.R. graphic sheet should include
   1. Accurately recorded T.P.R. (at least twice daily)
   2. Daily weights if indicated
   3. Intake and output—24-hour summary
   4. Indication of bowel habits

C. B.P. graphic sheet should include
   1. Clearly recorded times and dates
   2. Accurate B.P., pulse, and respiration recordings
   3. C.V.P., specific gravity, and frequent temperature measurements, if indicated

D. Medication sheet should include
   1. Properly dated columns
   2. Accurately and clearly indicated drug—name, dosage, route, time
   3. All injection sites
   4. "DC" written after final dose
   5. Proper notation of withheld medications
   6. Signature of person giving medications

E. Admission note information should include
   1. Time, date, mode of transportation, age, religion
   2. Temperature, pulse, respiration, blood pressure, height and weight
   3. Description of dentures and possession of eyeglasses, contact lens, hearing aids
   4. Signature of person who admits patient
   5. List of medications in patient's possession and disposition of these
   6. Allergies
   7. Deformities, bruises, prostheses, open wounds, or scars
   8. Diet requirements, preadmission diet
   9. Orientation of patient to hospital unit
   10. Time house staff notified
   11. Professional nursing assessment summary, which should include
       a. Patient's stated reason for admission
       b. Physical appearance
       c. Physical handicaps
       d. Names of medications patient has been taking or reasons if names are not known
       e. History and understanding of illness
       f. Reaction to illness and hospitalization
       g. Pertinent information on activities of home care and personal care

h. Nursing actions taken

F. Nurses' bedside sheet should include notes concerning
  1. Specific times for each entry
  2. All nursing interventions and observations
  3. Reasons for p.r.n. and stat drugs
  4. Medical and nursing ministrations
  5. Patient's reaction to nursing and medical ministrations
  6. Signs and symptoms displayed by patient
  7. Any further comment that communicates patient information to the next shift (each shift must chart)
  8. Signature, with title, for all statements
  9. Date and midnight
  10. Discharge note should include the time, mode, and a summary of information given to the patient and family for home care, names of medications sent with the patient, identification of the person who came for the patient, and the nurse's signature

G. Diabetic sheets (spot and/or fractional) should include
  1. Date, time, results of urine analysis for glucose and acetone
  2. Total amount of urine for each fractional and/or spot check
  3. Amount and kind of insulin
  4. Specific site of each injection
  5. Weight

H. Intravenous sheet should include
  1. Date
  2. Time, noting A.M. or P.M., and initials of person starting the infusion
  3. Type, amount of fluid, and added medications clearly written
  4. Amount absorbed, time discontinued
  5. Pertinent information, such as problems of administration or absorption, in *comment* column

Nursing care index follows.

Nursing care index—nursing record

Unit 10-S Date 11/20/73 Time 2 P.M.

Patient audit no. 1 Patient classification 3

Initials of member of committee D. W.

DEFINITION: Each item must be considered in relation to presence, relevance, and accuracy. Accurate or complete is here interpreted to mean that the information is correct, comprehensive, and written as indicated by the nursing care standards for the nursing records and the hospital procedures for the nursing records.

	YES	NO	COMMENT
A. Identification			
1. Are the patient's name and room number on the chart folder?	√		
2. Are all nursing chart forms labeled with the patient's first and last name and room number?	√		
3. Are allergy precautions noted accurately on the front of the chart?		√	*Allergic to Demerol (not noted)*
B. T.P.R. graphic sheet			
1. Are T.P.R.s recorded accurately?	√		
2. Are daily weights recorded?			
3. Are the I & O summaries accurately recorded?	√		
4. Are bowel habits indicated daily?	√		
C. B.P. graphic sheet			
1. Are vital signs recorded accurately?		√	*Missing 11/15 (9 p.m.)*
2. Are C.V.P.s, specific gravities, and temperatures that are recorded more frequently than every 4 hours accurately recorded?			
D. Medication			
1. Are columns dated, discontinued drugs noted, signatures present?	√		
2. Are drugs accurately written with dosage, route, time, and site of injection?		√	*Site missing 11/16*
3. Are withheld medications circled and an appropriate remark written in the nurses' notes?			

	YES	NO	COMMENT
E. Admission note			
1. Is all information filled in accurately?			*Admitted on other floor*
2. Are admission notes signed properly?			
3. Is there evidence that the patient's immediate needs were assessed by a registered nurse within the first hour?			
4. Is section on admission assessment completed?			
5. Is there a pertinent professional nursing assessment summary?			
F. Nurses' bedside notes			
1. Are dates and specific times indicated with comments for each shift, followed by signatures with titles?	√		
2. Are pertinent observations and communications recorded?	√		
3. Are treatments recorded accurately?	√		
4. Are nursing interventions recorded accurately?	√		
5. Is there evidence that the effectiveness of care has been evaluated?	√		
G. Diabetic sheet			
1. Is all pertinent information concerning test included?			
2. Are kind, amount, and site of injection of insulin clearly indicated and followed by signature?			
H. Intravenous sheets			
1. Are starting dates, times, signatures, and bottle numbers accurate?			
2. Are amounts, types, and additives accurate?			
3. Are completion dates, times, amounts absorbed, signatures, and comments accurate?			

Number of *yes* answers 11

Number of *no* answers 3

Total answered 14

CHAPTER 3

Information specific to practice of nursing–examples of procedures for self-directed learning

CONSTRUCTS IN NURSING

Various constructs seem to be essential both to the success with which specific groups function and to the success of individual members of the group. For professional nurses, such constructs include the philosophy, organizational chart, and goals, the dress code, and the conceptual framework of nursing.

Philosophy

The philosophy of a nursing service gives direction to thinking and actions of employees of the department. The philosophy implies whether or not there is commitment to principles of Christianity and to the rights of others. The new graduate must know the philosophy, since it will have an effect on her behavior.

In almost all cases the philosophy of a nursing service department indicates that the nursing service unit has an obligation to minister to the diverse needs of the patient—physical, psychological, spiritual, and economic. It also has a duty toward the patient's relatives—to treat them with kindness and to keep them informed regarding the progress of the patient.

Organizational chart

It is necessary that the department have an effective organization, providing centralization of authority as well as fixed responsibility (Fig. 1). Functions and relationships of each department and the members thereof should be precisely and clearly defined.

Goals

Nursing service goals or objectives must be identified and written by members of nursing administration and nursing staff. These may be formulated by a com-

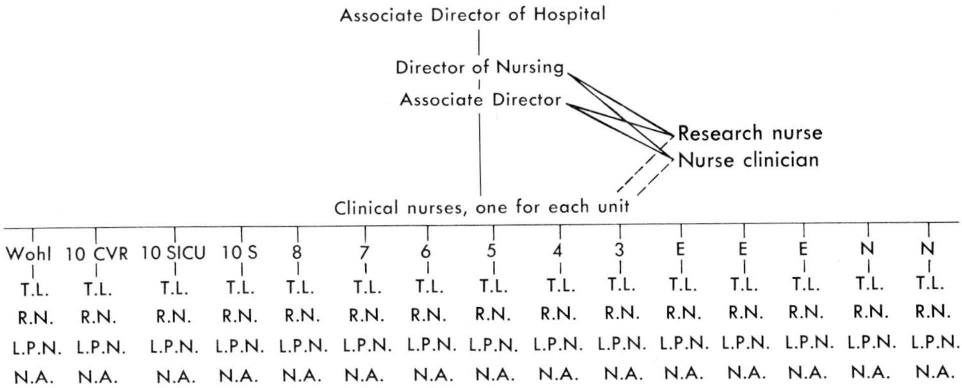

Bed capacity – 295

Staffing

R.N. staff – 115
L.P.N. staff – 92
N.A. staff – 55

Fig. 1. Organizational chart for department of nursing service.

mittee but should be approved by the nursing administration and staff. Among the goals of nursing service are the following:

1. To provide nursing care as established by the standards of nursing care adopted by the department of nursing.
2. To provide nursing service in full accordance with the policies and philosophy of the hospital.
3. To provide an environment conducive to self-development.
4. To engage in a continuing program of research for the improvement of nursing care.

Dress code

Each person is a product of the time and society in which he lives. Our behavior is influenced, and we influence the behavior of others by our dress and appearance. At this point in time, the factor of dress and appearance is a very controversial subject. Preferences and attention to dress and grooming differ among individuals. For this reason it would seem advisable that members of the nursing department establish a dress code that is acceptable to the majority of the members. Input into revision of the dress code should be ongoing. The items listed here are often included.

1. Caps and school pins will be worn at the discretion of the individual.
2. Pantsuits may be worn; however, the suit must be of regulation type, having a fingertip-length smock top. Only all white will be worn.
3. Length of white uniform may be mini, midi, or any length between but neither micro-mini nor maxi.

4. White shoes and hose will be worn.
5. Hair must be short or tied back with a narrow white ribbon, cord, rubber band, or hair clasp.
6. Name pins and university identification badges must be worn at all times.
7. Only tiny earrings for pierced ears may be worn.

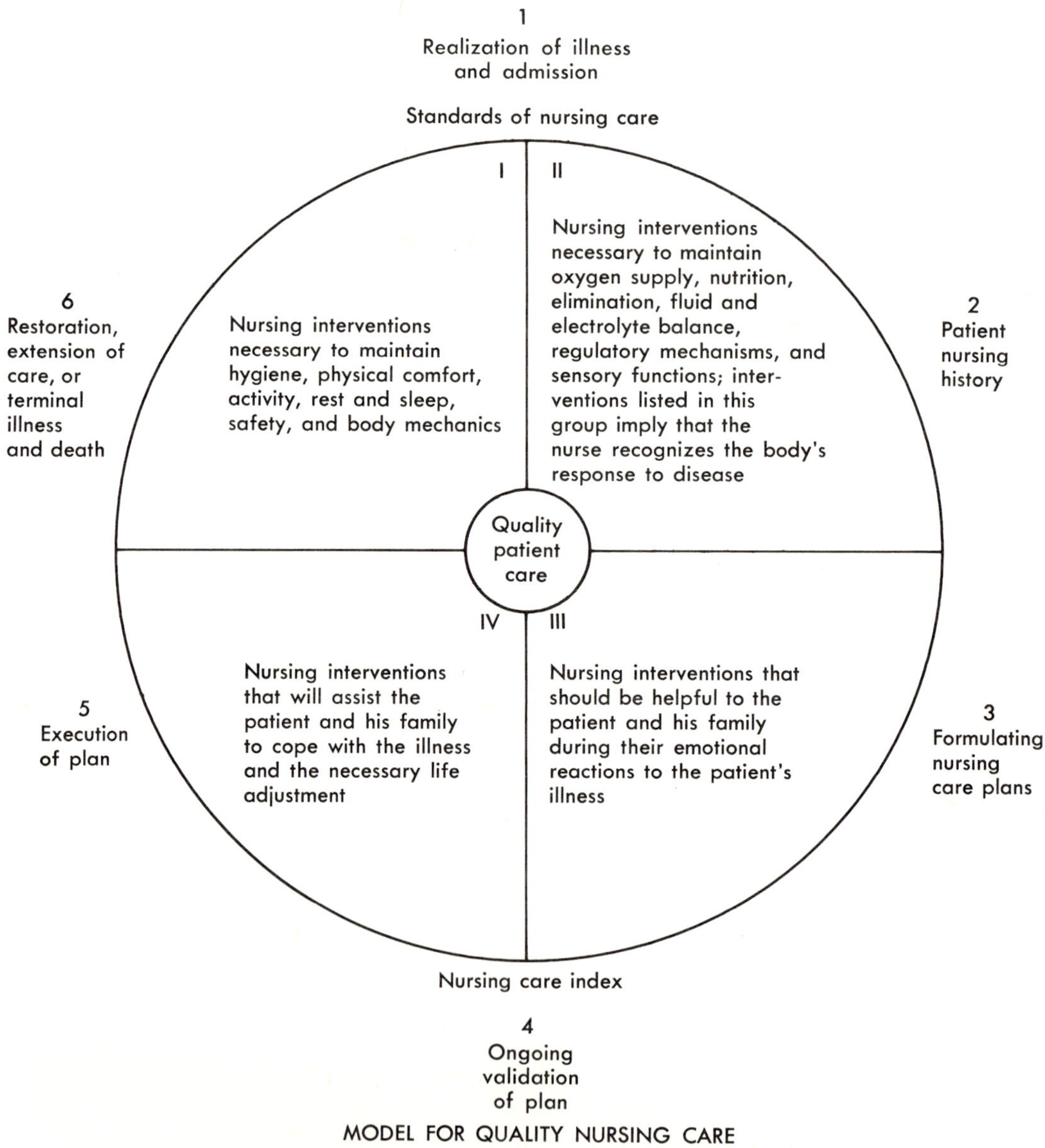

Fig. 2. Conceptual famework for activities of the department of nursing is "adaptation." The tool for action in the department of nursing is the accepted standards of nursing care.

8. Male personnel may wear conventional shoes and socks, with white pants and shirt.
9. Sweaters may be of any solid color, cardigan only.

Conceptual framework of nursing

The total nursing process can be expressed in the form of a model (Fig. 2), which will assist the nurse in perceiving the nursing process as a whole.

JOB SPECIFICATION

Clinical nurse

PURPOSE: To assist in the planning, organizing, and directing of nursing practice in accordance with the department's philosophy of nursing. To be responsible for one nursing unit.

QUALIFICATIONS:

A. Professional
   1. Is graduate of a recognized school of nursing and currently registered in the state where hospital is located.
   2. Has baccalaureate degree in nursing and at least two years of clinical experience or has five years of clinical experience with two years in a leadership position.
   3. Participates in continuing education programs.
   4. Holds membership in the American Nurses' Association.

B. Personal
   1. Is mature, poised, and capable of exercising independent judgment.
   2. Has ability to work effectively with others.

LINE OF AUTHORITY: Is responsible to the director of nursing service.

RESPONSIBILITIES:

A. Planning
   1. Participates in developing nursing goals in keeping with the organization's philosophy and objectives.
   2. Makes rounds with nursing personnel, administrators, and physicians to evaluate patient care.
   3. Assists in the development of standards of nursing care.
   4. Assures that the nursing unit is operating efficiently and effectively, co-operating with other hospital departments.
   5. Assumes responsibility for staffing of respective areas.
   6. Reviews all incident reports to identify problem areas for correction.
   7. Collaborates with the nurse clinicians and staff development instructors to identify staff and patient needs and to develop educational programs.

B. Organizing
   1. Confers with the director or the associate director of nursing service concerning interdepartmental and intradepartmental communication and problem solving.
   2. Participates in problem solving related to interdepartmental and intra-

departmental activities as delegated by the director of nursing service.
3. Cooperates with instructors from professional and technical schools of nursing to enhance student learning.

C. Directing and controlling
1. Communicates weekly with all nursing personnel, both to understand the problems of the units and to inform the nursing personnel of the hospital's goals, progress toward goals, and other significant information concerning the organization.
2. Participates in analysis and evaluation of each nursing unit's management and implements recommendations formalized by the Nursing Management Committee.
3. Assists in investigating complaints or expressions of dissatisfaction related to the practice of nursing.
4. Initiates the appropriate actions necessary to correct nursing problems.
5. Interprets hospital policies and supervises the implementation of the policies.
6. Participates in the implementation of the standards of nursing care.
7. Disciplines line nursing personnel in accordance with hospital policies.
8. Confers with team leaders concerning all information essential for continuity of patient care.
9. Directs and counsels all team leaders.
10. Reviews all requests for vacation, change of status, or leave of absence; all evaluations; all terminations.
11. Delegates responsibilities to team leaders.
12. Evaluates line nursing personnel on a yearly basis.

D. Teaching
1. Does incidental teaching of all personnel in their assigned areas.
2. Gives orientation and inservice instruction to the personnel in her assigned area. The orientation should not include close supervision but being available to help when a new professional feels the need for assistance.
3. Plans and directs continuing education for the personnel in her area.

Staff nurse/Team leader

PURPOSE:

A. To give skilled bedside care to patients according to their individual needs, including administration of medications and special treatments

B. To direct and supervise the care given by nonprofessional personnel

QUALIFICATIONS:

A. Professional and personal
1. Must be currently licensed by state to practice professional nursing.
2. Must show evidence of interest in continuous professional growth.
3. Must believe in the philosophy of team nursing and have confidence in her ability as a leader.

4. Must be able to apply scientific principles to problem solving and to planning, providing, and evaluating nursing care.
5. Must have a baccalaureate degree in nursing or be working toward it.

LINE OF AUTHORITY: Is responsible to clinical nurse or supervisor.

DUTIES:

A. General
   1. Knows standards of patient care established for hospital.
   2. Demonstrates an awareness of the total nursing needs of the patient and is responsible for seeing that they are met. Plans with the nursing team ways to meet these patient needs.
   3. Participates in the administration of nursing service by directing, supervising, and assisting the nonprofessional personnel in giving patient care.
   4. Participates in institutes, workshops, and research programs for the improvement of patient care and administration.
   5. Promotes a climate conducive to learning for both personnel and students.

B. Specific
   1. Attends change-of-shift report.
   2. Counts narcotics with nurse from previous shift.
   3. Visits all patients on team; makes adjustment of assignment according to the employees' abilities and patients' needs; also gives clarification report.
   4. Administers medications and manages fluid therapy.
   5. Confers with nurse clinician and/or supervisor about any problem.
   6. Confers with nurse clinician about nursing care management.
   7. Immediately visits after all new admissions, observes patient conditions and reactions of patient to hospitalization, and checks for identification band. Is responsible for writing an admission assessment in the nursing progress notes.
   8. Confers with service supervisor regarding patient transfer—whether within, onto, or off the unit.
   9. Plans and coordinates patient discharge.
   10. Reports to service supervisor any problem regarding housekeeping, maintenance, adequate supplies, scheduling of diagnostic procedures, or clarification of physicians' orders.
   11. Plans, directs, and assists with bedside nursing care given to patients in her assigned area.
   12. Makes rounds as frequently as necessary for the purposes of observing, assessing, and meeting patient needs and supervising or assisting personnel for whom she is responsible.
   13. Instructs and checks all patients before they go to surgery and completes the preoperative checklist.
   14. Visits all postoperative patients immediately on their return to unit.
   15. Sees all emergency cases immediately, reports all incidental mishaps or

injuries to the nursing supervisor, and makes out a single copy of incident report.

16. Makes rounds with house staff, professor, and private physicians.
17. Calls member of house staff as necessary to meet needs of a patient and informs him of any changes in the patient's condition that he should be aware of.
18. Assists physicians as required in administration of treatments, in performing diagnostic tests, in changing dressings, etc.
19. Calls the chaplain at the patient's or family's request or if a change in a patient's condition indicates.
20. Notifies clinical nurse and/or supervisor about any unusual problems or serious changes in any patient's condition.
21. Examines transcriptions of doctors' orders, for accuracy.
22. Conducts daily team conference.
23. Receives report from personnel on team as to care they have given and each patient's condition.
24. Charts all observations and changes in conditions on the appropriate patient's chart.

NURSING UNIT 24-HOUR REPORT

List all new admissions scheduled (name, room, diagnosis, other pertinent information)
List all critically ill patients (name, room, diagnosis, other pertinent information)
List all pertinent information pertaining to patient, family, visitor, employee, or nursing unit problems

UNIT		DATE
DAY CENSUS*	EVENING CENSUS*	NIGHT CENSUS*
*Each team leader to sign	*Each team leader to sign	*Each team leader to sign

Fig. 3

25. Daily checks nursing Kardex for thoroughness, accuracy, and legibility and for continuity of patient care.
26. Checks patient charts daily for accuracy and completeness.
27. Makes assignments (patient care and functional) for the following day by 2:30 P.M.
28. Gives report to charge nurse on next shift and count narcotics with her.
29. Keeps records and submits reports as follows:
    a. Completes an anecdotal record on each team member twice weekly.
    b. Completes nursing unit 24-hour report (Fig. 3) by 2 P.M., 10 P.M., 6 A.M.
    c. Completes patient condition record (Fig. 4, p. 74).

C. Additional duties of 3 to 11 nurse
1. Secures operative permit and urine specimens from newly admitted patients.
2. Instructs patients regarding diagnostic or operative procedures.
3. Sees that radios and televisions are toned down by 9 P.M. and turned off by 10 P.M.
4. Sees that patients are properly prepared for sleep and that all utility areas are clean and orderly before personnel leave for the night.
5. Updates patient condition sheet.
6. Sees that all visitors are off the unit by 9 P.M. unless the patient's condition warrants someone staying. Notifies security guards if visitors without permission remain on unit after 9 P.M., after they have been asked to leave.

D. Additional duties of 11 to 7 nurse
1. Completes condition sheet for night supervisor.
2. Checks diet list.
3. Checks patients who are n.p.o. for surgery or diagnostic tests.
4. Makes rounds, seeing every patient every hour.

Student nurse

PURPOSE: Under close and frequent guidance of the professional nurse, the student nurse performs specific duties of patient care.

QUALIFICATIONS:

A. School and experience
1. Must be classified as at least a first semester junior in an accredited school of nursing or equivalent (having had at least two nursing practicum courses).

B. Personal
1. Must be well groomed, friendly, industrious, punctual, and reliable and demonstrate outstanding ability in her job performance.

LINE OF AUTHORITY: Reports to team leader or charge nurse regarding patient care. Confers with nursing supervisor regarding problems.

DUTIES:

A. General

1. Gives nursing care to patients according to job description and standards of nursing care.
2. Assists in maintaining order and cleanliness within the unit.

B. Specific

1. Performs direct patient care.
    a. Assists with admission.
    b. Gives bath—tub, bed, or shower.
    c. Gives oral hygiene.
    d. Grooms patient in regard to hair, nails, and shaving when indicated.
    e. Gives simple skin care—lotion to back and to pressure areas; special skin care to dry skin areas.
    f. Positions patients.
        (1) Turns and positions bed patients with simple supports.
        (2) Assists in transporting patients.
        (3) Gives range of motion exercises as assigned.
    g. Prepares patients for meals. Assists and feeds patients when necessary.
        (1) Administers between-meal nourishment.
        (2) Forces or restricts fluids as directed.
    h. Assists with preoperative and postoperative care of patients.
    i. Assists with transfer and discharge of patients.
    j. Assists with postmortem care—transports body to morgue.
    k. Assists patients with coughing and deep breathing exercise when assigned.
    l. Assists with sitz bath.
    m. Gives perineal care.
    n. Assists team members with patients as needed.
    o. Cares for patients in isolation.
    p. Cares for patients on Stryker frame.
    q. Cares for patients receiving oxygen therapy, traction, continuous bladder irrigation, nasal-gastric suctioning, Hemovac, intravenous therapy, etc.
    r. Applies ice packs or Aqua-matic pads and assists with hypothermia mattress, flotation pads, air mattress, etc.
    s. Suctions patients and gives tube feedings to patients—under the supervision of the team leader.
2. Provides a comfortable and safe environment.
    a. Changes bed linen of each patient daily and changes linen as necessary to keep patient dry.
    b. Adjusts bed, side rails, and call light for patient's convenience.
    c. Gives and removes bedpan, urinal, emesis basin. Keeps these utensils clean and stores them in proper place.
    d. Maintains environment for patient's comfort.
    e. Passes fresh water and places it within patient's reach.
    f. Does assigned housekeeping duties.

3. Helps with treatments and collects specimens.
   a. Gives simple enemas—cleansing and Fleets.
   b. Collects simple specimens.
      (1) Urine—simple, double-voided, fractional, specimens for culture and sensitivity, and 24-hour specimens.
      (2) Stools.
      (3) Sputum—culture and sensitivity, 24-hour, and cytology.
   c. Assists physician with minor procedures and physical examinations.
4. Performs (or measures) and charts the following.
   a. Admits new patient and completes first part of admission form.
   b. Takes and charts T.P.R.—temperatures (oral, rectal, and axillary); pulse (radial); and respirations—also records blood pressure and weight.
   c. Computes intake and output—on basis of oral intake, simple Foley bag collection, and Gomco suction.
   d. Records double-voided specimen and fractional urine specimens.
   e. Determines specific gravity.
   f. Charts patient observations and nursing care interventions if the student has been instructed to chart during her nursing education. The team leader is expected to review the student's charting and note any additional comments.
5. Communications.
   a. Reports problems, changes, or questions to team leader or charge nurse.
   b. Attends clarification report and participates actively in team conference.
   c. Makes frequent rounds on all assigned patients, noting condition, requests, identification, and environment. NOTE: On the 11 to 7 shift, rounds are to be made every 30 minutes, noting condition and environment of assigned patients.
   d. All nursing care given by a student nurse is directly supervised by the team leader or charge nurse. If the team leader is unaware of the student nurse's previous nursing experience or nursing capabilities, she should observe the student's performance of nursing duties until she feels the student can satisfactorily perform each task.

Licensed practical nurse

PURPOSE: Under the direction and supervision of the professional nurse, gives simple and complex care to all types of patients.

QUALIFICATIONS:

A. School and experience
   1. Must be high school graduate, have certificate from approved school for practical nurses, and be registered in the state.

B. Personal

1. Must be at least 18 years of age and have some appreciation of the responsibility of her work.

LINE OF AUTHORITY: Reports to and is supervised by team leader, charge nurse, or supervisor regarding patient care. Confers with nurse in charge on patient problems, any uncertainty in methods of procedure, and all incidents that might affect patients, personnel, or visitors adversely.

DUTIES:

A. General
   1. Gives bedside nursing care to all types of patients according to standards of nursing care.
   2. Assists in maintaining order and cleanliness within the unit.

B. Specific
   1. Performs direct patient care.
      a. Admits patients.
      b. Gives bath—bed, tub, or shower.
      c. Gives oral hygiene.
      d. Grooms patients in regard to hair, nails, and shaving when indicated.
      e. Gives skin care, including decubitus care.
      f. Turns and positions patients in bed and chair.
      g. Gives range of motion exercises as indicated.
      h. Ambulates patients as ordered.
      i. Prepares patients for meals. Assists and feeds patients when necessary.
         (1) Administers between-meal nourishment.
         (2) Forces or restricts fluids as ordered.
      j. Does preoperative and postoperative care of patients.
      k. Assists patients with coughing and deep breathing exercise when ordered.
      l. Does postmortem care and transports body to morgue.
      m. Cares for patients having oxygen therapy, monitors, respirator, peritoneal dialysis, Stryker frame, hypothermia, Hemovac, traction, prostheses, flotation pad, Aqua-matic pad, air mattress, chest tube, continuous bladder irrigation, etc.
      n. Applies dressings, bandages, slings, binders, Ace bandages, and elastic stockings when ordered.
      o. Cares for patients in isolation.
      p. Assists team members with patients as needed.
      q. Answers all lights promptly.
   2. Provides a comfortable and safe environment.
      a. Changes bed linen of each patient daily and changes linen as necessary to keep patient dry.
      b. Adjusts bed, side rails, and call light for patient's convenience.
      c. Applies restraints as ordered.

d. Gives and removes bedpan, urinal, and emesis basin. Keeps these utensils clean and stores them in proper place.
e. Maintains environment for patient's comfort.
f. Passes fresh water and places it within patient's reach.
g. Does assigned housekeeping duties.

3. Does treatments, collects specimens, and charts.
   a. Gives enemas, douches, perineal care, and sitz baths; also inserts colon tubes, irrigates colostomies, and changes colostomy dressing.
   b. Collects specimens—urine, stool, and sputum.
   c. Does spot checks and fractional and specific gravity measurements.
   d. Catheterizes and does Foley catheter irrigation.
   e. Gives ice bags and hot water bottles only as ordered.
   f. Irrigates nasal-gastric tubes.
   g. Gives tube feedings and gastrostomy feeding at the direction of the nurse.
   h. Performs nasal, oral, and tracheostomy suction and care as needed.
   i. Takes temperatures (oral, rectal, axillary); pulses (apical, radial, pedal); respirations; blood pressure and central venous pressure (C.V.P.) measurements.
   j. Computes and records intake and output.
   k. Gives medication only after a period of instruction and observation.
   l. Assists physician with procedures and physical examinations.
   m. Discontinues intravenous fluids at the direction of the nurse.
   n. Admits, discharges, and assists with transferring patients.
   o. Charts pertinent notes according to standards.
   p. Assists with cardiopulmonary resuscitation (CPR).
4. Communications.
   a. Listens to change-of-shift report when assigned to administer medications.
   b. Checks assignment with nurse in charge.
   c. Attends clarification report and participates actively in team conference.
   d. Knows the responsibilities of a team member.
   e. Makes frequent rounds on all patients, noting condition, requests, identification, and environment, and reports to nurse when indicated.

Nursing assistant I

PURPOSE: Under close and frequent guidance of the professional nurse, the nursing assistant performs specific, uncomplicated duties of patient care.

QUALIFICATIONS:

A. School and experience
   1. Is a high school graduate.
   2. Is at least 18 years of age with one year of work experience.
   3. Has completed a specified period of time in some recognized program.

4. Demonstrates some exceptional ability to meet job requirements.

B. Personal

1. Must be well groomed, friendly, and industrious and show some desire to advance in her job.

LINE OF AUTHORITY: Reports to team leader or charge nurse regarding patient care. Confers with supervisor regarding problems.

DUTIES:

A. General

1. Gives nursing care to patients according to job description and standards of nursing care.
2. Assists in maintaining order and cleanliness within the unit.

B. Specific

1. Performs direct patient care.
   a. Assists with admission.
   b. Gives bath—tub, bed, or shower.
   c. Gives oral hygiene.
   d. Grooms patient in regard to hair, nails, and shaving when indicated.
   e. Gives simple skin care—lotion to back and to pressure areas; special skin care to dry skin areas.
   f. Positions patients.
      (1) Turns and positions bed patients with simple supports.
      (2) Assists in transporting patients.
      (3) Positions patients in chair.
      (4) Gives range of motion exercise as assigned.
   g. Prepares patients for meals. Assists and feeds patients when necessary.
      (1) Administers between-meals nourishment.
      (2) Forces or restricts fluids as directed.
   h. Assists with preoperative and postoperative care of patients.
   i. Assists with transferring and discharge of patients.
   j. Assists with postmortem care—transports body to morgue.
   k. Assists patient with coughing and deep breathing exercise when assigned.
   l. Assists with sitz bath.
   m. Gives perineal care.
   n. Assists team members with patients as needed.
2. Provides a comfortable and safe environment.
   a. Changes bed linen of each patient daily and changes linen as necessary to keep patient dry.
   b. Adjusts bed, side rails, call light for patient's convenience.
   c. Gives and removes bedpan, urinal, emesis basin. Keeps these utensils clean and stores them in proper place.
   d. Maintains environment for patient's comfort.
   e. Passes fresh water and places within patient's reach.
   f. Does assigned housekeeping duties.

3. Helps with treatments and collects specimens.
   a. Gives simple enemas—cleansing and Fleets.
   b. Collects simple specimens.
      (1) Urine—simple, double-voided and fractional specimens, for culture and sensitivity, and 24-hour specimens.
      (2) Stools.
      (3) Sputum—culture and sensitivity, 24-hour, and cytology.
   c. Applies ice packs or Aqua-matic pads and assists with hypothermia mattress, flotation pads, air mattress, etc.
   d. Assists physician with minor procedures and physical examinations.
4. Performs and charts as follows.
   a. Admits new patient and completes first part of admission form.
   b. Takes and charts T.P.R.—temperatures (oral, rectal, and axillary); pulse (radial); and respirations—also records blood pressure and weight.
   c. Computes intake and output—on basis of oral intake, simple Foley bag collection, Gomco suction.
5. Communications.
   a. Reports problems, changes, or questions to team leader or charge nurse.
   b. Attends clarification report and participates actively in team conference.
   c. Makes frequent rounds on all assigned patients, noting condition, requests, identification, and environment. NOTE: On 11 to 7 shift, rounds are to be made every 30 minutes, noting condition and environment of assigned patients.
   d. Answers all lights promptly.

Nursing assistant II

PURPOSE: Under close and frequent guidance of the professional nurse, the nursing assistant performs specific, uncomplicated duties of patient care.

QUALIFICATIONS:

A. School and experience
   1. Is a high school graduate.
   2. Is at least 18 years of age with one year of experience in this hospital.
   3. Has completed a specified period of time in some recognized program.
   4. Demonstrates some exceptional ability to meet job requirements.

B. Personal
   1. Must be well groomed, friendly, industrious, punctual, and reliable and demonstrate outstanding ability in her job performance.

LINE OF AUTHORITY: Reports to team leader or charge nurse regarding patient care. Confers with supervisor regarding problems.

DUTIES:

A. General
   1. Gives nursing care to patients according to job description and standards of nursing care.

2. Assists in maintaining order and cleanliness within the unit.

B. Specific
   1. Performs all duties in the scope of nursing assistant I, with the following additional duties in direct patient care.
      a. Cares for patients in isolation.
      b. Cares for patients on Stryker frame.
      c. Cares for patients receiving oxygen therapy, traction, continuous bladder irrigation, nasal-gastric suctioning, Hemovac, intravenous therapy, etc.
      d. Cares for newborns and assists with care of patients in labor and delivery.
      e. Applies slings, binders, Ace bandages, and elastic stockings.
   2. Obtains and charts the following.
      a. Double-voided specimen and fractional urine specimen.
      b. Measurements of specific gravity.

POSITION DESCRIPTION

Service supervisor/Unit manager

A. Definition of the position
   The service supervisor, or unit manager, is directly responsible and accountable for the nonnursing functions on the patient floors.

B. General qualifications
   1. Educational requirements
      a. High school graduation the minimal requirement.
      b. Two or more years of college preparation desirable, with concentration in business administration preferred.
   2. Experience requirements
      a. One year, or preferably more, of successful experience in a management position in a hospital or other health care facility desirable.
      b. Acceptable reference, based on previous employment or schooling.
   3. Age—21 to 50 years.
   4. Sex—nondiscriminatory.
   5. Race or national origin—nondiscriminatory.

C. Personal requirements
   1. Good grooming and appearance.
   2. Understanding and practice of ethical and professional conduct.
   3. Good memory for details.
   4. Ability to work under pressure and take criticism.
   5. Ability to organize and complete work.
   6. Habit of speaking correctly, quietly, audibly, in a courteous and friendly manner.
   7. Ability to work effectively with others.
   8. Ability to communicate effectively verbally and in writing.
   9. Ability to assume management responsibilities.
   10. Self-motivation.

D. Health requirements
   1. Good physical and mental health as evidenced by a good attendance record and good attitude.
   2. Annual chest x-ray film and physical examination.

E. Position responsibilities
   1. Responsible to the director of the patient service department and through him to the associate director of the hospital.
   2. Held responsible and accountable for the work performance of the unit secretary assigned to his/her area.
   3. Expected to know hospital policies as they relate to nursing division functions and to interpret them in concert with the philosophy and objectives of the organization.
   4. Responsible and accountable for disaster preparedness on the nursing division and for maintenance of a fire-safe and accident-free environment.

F. Coverage
   1. Responsible and accountable for his/her assigned area on a 24-hour basis.
   2. Required to rotate on a weekend coverage schedule. In addition to other specific duties during weekend coverage, the service supervisor must coordinate to assure full coverage by unit secretaries and transporters. On holidays and exceptionally busy weekends, 2 service supervisors are assigned to cover the hospital. One is assigned to medical floors and the other to surgical floors, but they may realign to satisfy the needs of the hospital.

G. Responsible and accountable for the preparation and maintenance of an acceptable patient environment
   1. Makes daily rounds in patient rooms to assure cleanliness and completeness.
   2. Makes daily or weekly rounds with assistant director of nursing service assigned to the area.
      a. Determines patient needs that are not being met because of shortage of supplies and/or equipment.
      b. Determines patient complaints.
      c. Weighs and assesses alternative solutions.
         (1) Uses information gathered to determine best alternative.
         (2) Implements best alternative.
      d. Checks patient name bands daily to assure completeness and accuracy of records.
   3. Assures that patient discharges are handled promptly and properly.
      a. Telephones admitting department promptly when discharge order is written so that information available to admitting office for use in room assignment is current and accurate at all times.
      b. Assesses with resident, on a daily basis, the list of patients who may be discharged the next day.
      c. Discusses with the patient who is to be discharged the requirement of meeting the 11:00 A.M. deadline.

d. Follows discharge procedure carefully.
e. Works with physicians to assure that discharge orders are written on a timely basis to allow meeting the 11:00 A.M. deadline as consistently as possible.

H. Responsible and accountable for the timely and accurate completion of the transfer procedure
1. Assigns rooms after appropriate consultation with nurse team leader and physician.
2. Telephones admitting department promptly when a patient is to be transferred, giving full and accurate details, so that the information available there is current at all times.
3. Assures that all patient belongings are transferred with the patient.

I. Responsible and accountable for coordination of assignment of patient rooms
1. Makes every effort to assign male rooms next to male rooms, and female next to female, when bathrooms are shared.
2. Assigns rooms in accordance with compatibility regarding sex, age, and medical diagnosis.
3. Assures that patients who are critically ill are placed as close to nursing station as possible. These patients may not meet requirements for placement in an intensive care area, or they may be patients for whom no space is available in the units.

J. Responsible for release of body from nursing division
1. Notifies physician.
2. Notifies family. This duty is best left with the physician, but the service supervisor can perform this function. It shall *not* be delegated to the unit secretary.
3. Notifies admitting department promptly of death of patients, so that the information available in the admitting office, for room assignment, is current at all times.
4. Notifies switchboard.
5. Orders morgue pack from central service.
6. Directs or personally effects the removal of the body to the morgue.
7. Completes discharge procedure carefully.

K. Responsible for inspection of all new makeups and assurance that room is acceptable for next patient before his arrival
1. Coordinates all problems associated with room makeups with housekeeping personnel.
2. Notifies admitting department of any problems that may cause delay in acceptable room assignment.

L. Responsible and accountable for processing physicians' orders
1. Checks daily to see that orders have been correctly transcribed.
2. Informs nurse team leader of new orders that may be of critical nature.
3. Checks with physician regarding any questionable orders.
4. Notifies physician and nurse of any errors made in transcription.
5. Gives a report to oncoming unit secretary regarding new orders and duties.

6. Confers with team leader and physician regarding up-to-dateness of orders.
7. Orients new house staff to floor protocol.
8. Assists unit secretary in interpreting orders.
9. Checks that daily blood work is ordered.
10. Assures proper use of Kardex.

M. Responsible for location and condition of patient's chart
1. Checks new charts to see that admission notes are filled out completely.
2. Checks daily to see that all new sheets have been stamped and charts are in order.
3. Locates missing charts.
4. Keeps old charts on floor for use of physician.
5. Organizes record and assures its completeness at time of discharge. Sends to medical records.
6. Checks charts daily to assure minimization to turnaround time for reporting results of patient testing.

N. Responsible for all supplies and equipment assigned and delivered to patient floor
1. Orders all stock medications (daily).
2. Orders all stock central service supplies (daily).
3. Orders weekly storeroom supplies according to ordering schedule.
4. Checks equipment on the unit and reports needed repairs.
5. Makes daily rounds of patient rooms to inspect for maintenance, cleanliness, and completeness of unit.
6. Reports the necessity for procuring equipment.
7. Keeps records of all supplies ordered by the unit.
8. Follows up on maintenance requests when performed.
9. Accounts for chargeable items used by patient.
10. Makes an inspection of needed linens twice daily and coordinates. Makes necessary adjustments.

O. Responsible for arranging periodic meetings with nurse team leader and resident physician to discuss and solve common problems
1. Provides useful management information.
2. Accepts suggestions for improvement in supply (equipment, delivery, and/or maintenance).
3. Interprets hospital policy.
4. Discusses equipment problems and reviews team member responsibilities.

P. Responsible for dietary needs of the unit
1. Maintains acceptable stock of patient nourishments.
2. Assures that unit secretary telephones accurate information regarding hold, n.p.o., late trays, etc. to proper personnel on a timely basis.
3. Coordinates meal delivery with appropriate members of food service management to assure effective and efficient service to patients.
4. Communicates unresolved problems up the organization.

Q. Responsible and accountable for assurance that the cardiopulmonary resuscitation cart is completely ready for the next emergency

1. Supervises to avoid borrowing from cart.
2. Provides additional floor stock of heavily used supplies to avoid abuse of cart system.
3. Observes routine checking of cart by inhalation therapy personnel. Communicates deviations from standard to chief inhalation therapist.
4. Assures that a form is available on the cart for use in listing medications and supplies used during arrest.
5. Checking emergency cart shall be considered a top priority of each working day.

R. Responsible and accountable for the direct supervision of the unit secretaries assigned to the area
   1. Assures daily coverage by coordinating to resolve deviations.
   2. Participates in screening unit secretary applicants for replacement in respective areas.
   3. Assumes responsibility for enacting corrective action policy or termination of unit secretary when warranted.
   4. Assists in orientation and training of new unit secretary assigned to respective area.
   5. Holds periodic conferences with individual secretary or with group to improve morale, correct poor work habits, and teach new procedures.
   6. Writes performance appraisal report for unit secretaries routinely assigned to respective area.

S. Responsible for interpretation and enforcement of hospital policies on the patient floors

T. Responsible for supply, distribution, completion, and disposition of the following forms, and others
   1. Leave of absence (pass).
   2. Surgical consent form.
   3. Against medical advice.
   4. Infection control.
   5. Consent for autopsy.
   6. Bequest of the body.

U. Responsible and accountable for the maintenance of unit bulletin boards, procedure and policy manuals with all pertinent notices

V. Responsible for transporting patients when transportation is not readily available

Unit secretary/Ward clerk

A. Definition of position

   A unit secretary, or ward clerk, performs duties under the general supervision of the service supervisor.

B. Qualifications
   1. Educational requirements—high school graduate.
   2. Age—19-50.
   3. Sex—nondiscriminatory.

4. Experience required.
   a. Minimum of one year of business experience desired.
   b. Good recommendations.
5. Personal requirements.
   a. Good grooming and appearance.
   b. Interest in hospital work.
   c. Habits of speaking correctly, quietly, and audibly and exhibiting a courteous friendly manner.
   d. Ability to work effectively with others.
   e. Ability to communicate effectively.
   f. Understanding and practice of ethical conduct.
   g. Accuracy and good memory for details.
   h. Ability to organize and complete work.
   i. Ability to work under pressure and take criticism—justified or otherwise.
6. Health requirements.
   a. Good physical and mental health as evidenced by a good work attendance record.
   b. To have a physical examination, including chest x-ray film, on a yearly basis.

C. Position responsibilities
1. Is responsible to the service supervisor and through him to the director, patient service department.
2. Has a thorough knowledge of duties.

D. Specific duties
1. Charts.
   a. Assembles charts on all patients.
   b. Fills in headings on charts.
   c. Adds new sheets to charts.
   d. Keeps charts in order at all times.
   e. Secures old charts for authorized personnel.
2. Transcribes orders.
   a. Systematically transcribes orders from patient's order sheet to Kardex.
   b. Initiates requisitions for diagnostic, consultative, and therapeutic departments.
   c. Refers pertinent information to nursing staff by means of a ticket.
3. Prepares requisitions.
   a. Initiates requisitions for the following areas.
      (1) Pharmacy. (3) Central service.
      (2) Dietary. (4) Linen.
4. Acts as receptionist.
   a. Directs visitors to patients.
   b. Directs hospital personnel to patients, charts, etc.
   c. Receives and transmits telephone communications.
   d. Distributes flowers and gifts left at nursing station.

5. Assists in admission of patients.
   a. Welcomes and escorts patient to room.
   b. Notifies appropriate personnel of new admission.
6. Aids in transfer and discharge of patients.
   a. Assists service supervisor with established transfer procedure.
7. Prepares daily census sheets.
8. Assists with receiving, distributing, and storing articles brought to floor.
9. Demonstrates awareness in the conservation of hospital supplies and equipment.
10. Maintains nursing station area in an orderly manner.

ORGANIZATION AND QUALITY NURSING CARE

Structural and organizational arrangements include the introduction of the nursing team—made up of a professional staff nurse who functions in the role of team leader and other professional staff nurses, licensed practical nurses, nurse assistants, and orderlies who function in the role of team members—with the team leader assuming responsibility for the provision of patient care in a circumscribed area. The clinical nurse "decentralizes" authority to the team leader to direct the activities of her team members. The clinical nurse is no longer the hub of the communication system, since team members communicate directly with the team leader instead of with the clinical nurse. The nursing unit is divided into team areas with a census of from 10 to 20 patients making it feasible and possible for one qualified team leader to effectively direct 2 to 5 team members in the actual execution of patient care. The team conference is introduced as a tool for the purpose of allowing the entire team to plan and evaluate patient care.

The team leader has the charged responsibility for synchronizing the abilities of her team members so that they can function effectively in a team relationship. Emphasis is placed on the ability of all participating in patient care to plan, administer, and evaluate patient care.

TEAM NURSING

Definition and description

Team nursing is a pattern of patient care that involves changes in the structural and organizational framework of the nursing unit and the deliberate introduction of the team concept for the stated aim of utilizing all levels of personnel to their fullest capacity in giving the best possible nursing care to patients.

Functions of the team leader

The team leader is a professional nurse. Her competence as a nurse practitioner is emphasized. As a participant in nursing care, she plans, directs, coordinates, controls, administers, and evaluates care given to a group of assigned patients. The team leader directly supervises and teaches members of the nursing team. She is responsible for providing preventive, therapeutic, palliative, and/or rehabilitative care for each patient. Her primary function is that of providing patient-centered care in the following ways.

A. Identifying patients' needs and the nursing problems—physical, spiritual, social, and psychological
   1. Possesses a knowledge and understanding of the physical, social, and biological sciences.
   2. Possesses skill in problem solving.

B. Interpreting nursing needs to co-workers and seeking their cooperation in planning
   1. Communicates directly with clinical nurse and team members.
   2. Provides for on-the-spot conferences with team members.
   3. Formulates and gives accurate reports.
   4. Formulates immediate and long-term objectives of nursing care.
   5. Develops an awareness of nursing responsibilities associated with the total medical care plan.

C. Formulating, with the team members, a nursing care plan for each patient and recording the plan of care

D. Distinguishing and delegating the many aspects of nursing care
   1. Evaluates the abilities of the members of the team. (See anecdotal records that follow.)
   2. Knows the background and experience of each team member.
   3. Keeps well informed about hospital policies regulating the activities of each member.
   4. Maintains personal contact with all patients in the team.
   5. Determines the *total* nursing needs.
   6. Delegates care to professional nurse, practical nurse, and the nursing assistant.

E. Directing and participating in nursing care
   1. Assumes the administrative responsibility for the assignment of patients.
   2. Provides direct supervision of the team.
   3. Participates in the administration of nursing care.
   4. Provides direction and guidance.
      a. On-the-spot teaching and assistance.
      b. Daily team conferences.
      c. Teaching by example.
   5. Recognizes and accepts the contribution made by each member of the team.
   6. Assists team members to evaluate performance.

F. Evaluating and recording the results of nursing care
   1. Determines the response of the patient to the nursing care—physical, social, spiritual, and psychological.
   2. Maintains a "progress record."
      a. Nurses' notes.
      b. Nursing care plan.

Ongoing evaluation is one of the responsibilities of the professional nurse. The following are examples.

Team leader anecdotal record—each shift

Name____________________Patient census____________________

Date____________________Total number of category 4 and 5 patients______

Team leader principles	YES	NO	SOMETIMES	COMMENTS
1. Receives an appropriate report from offgoing team leader.				
a. Utilizes the team leader worksheet and Kardex.				
b. Clarifies the report with offgoing team leader.				
2. Counts narcotics with offgoing and with oncoming team leader.				
3. If unable to account for missing narcotics, notifies the supervisor.				
4. Conducts clarification report, referring to the nursing care plan, for team members by walking-planning rounds within 1½ hours after arrival on duty.				
5. If unit is particularly busy, makes own rounds and then gives team members clarification report within 1½ hours after arrival on duty.				
6. Periodically makes rounds on team to assess needs of team members.				
a. Controls and directs work of team members.				
b. Recognizes learning needs of team members and teaches nursing skills and procedures when indicated.				
7. Periodically makes rounds on team to assess patients' needs.				
8. Makes rounds with physicians on the unit.				
9. Conducts an appropriate team conference every day.				
a. Informs team members of changes in patient conditions or any other changes occurring on the unit.				
b. Receives pertinent reports from team members.				
c. Develops a practical nursing care plan in accordance with the hospital's standards—for the Kardex.				

	YES	NO	SOMETIMES	COMMENTS
d. Utilizes the nursing history form in preparing the nursing care plan.				
e. Encourages team members' participation in developing the nursing care plan.				
f. Teaches team members during conference when indicated.				
g. Keeps Kardex and nursing care plan current.				
h. Updates record of last B.M. on patient's Kardex.				
10. Prepares census and condition sheet.				
11. Prepares nursing report for the nursing supervisor.				
12. Develops supervisory skills.				
a. Prepares anecdotal records concerning team members' performance—two a week.				
b. Counsels team members when nursing performance indicates it to be necessary.				
c. Praises team members when nursing performance indicates a commendation.				
13. Utilizes the nursing history form in writing the patient's admission assessment.				
14. Records in patient's chart a nursing assessment within 1 hour after patient's admission on the unit.				
15. Utilizes resources appropriately.				
a. Informs supervisor of unit problems.				
b. Informs nurse clinician of patients' needs when indicated.				
c. Informs physicians of patients' needs.				
d. Informs service supervisor and secretary of patients' and unit's needs.				
e. Notifies hospital chaplain and supervisor of critical patients, patients who arrest, or patients having unscheduled surgery—prior to that surgery—when secretary is unable to place calls.				

Continued.

	YES	NO	SOMETIMES	COMMENTS
16. Prepares nursing care assignments for the following day before leaving duty.				
a. Informs nursing office if there are too few or too many on nursing staff.				
b. Distributes the patients among her team members, considering the various patients' needs and team members' abilities.				
17. Conducts an appropriate change-of-shift report.				
a. Utilizes the tape recorder.				
b. Reports concise, accurate, and pertinent information.				
c. Utilizes the team leader worksheet and Kardex.				
d. Clarifies report with oncoming team leader if necessary.				
Charting 1. Charts pertinent nursing notes.				
2. Charts medications correctly.				
3. Utilizes the backs of pink medication cards (sites of injections) and white medication cards (pulses for Lanoxin).				
4. Circles a medication not given.				
5. Makes an appropriate nursing note for medication not given.				
6. Charts intravenous fluids and IV additives, transfusions, and albumin on the parenteral therapy sheet.				
7. Utilizes time tapes correctly on IV bottles.				
8. Checks that nursing personnel have charted correctly—T.P.R., vital signs, spot checks, I & O, weights, B.M.s.				
9. Charts for attendants.				
10. Reviews charting of ancillary personnel and adds additional information. **Professionalism**				
1. Reports to duty on time.				
2. Notifies nursing office 4 hours prior to duty time if unable to come to work or will be late.				

	YES	NO	SOMETIMES	COMMENTS
3. Attends physician lectures and conferences.				
4. Attends monthly nursing staff meetings.				
5. Responds positively to nursing service's requests—overtime and pulling to another division.				
6. Oversees environment (nursing conference room, patient area, and nursing station) to see that it is free of clutter.				
7. Is aware of own limitations and seeks assistance when needed.				
8. Relates with other team leaders; establishes a working relationship.				
9. Relates with team members; establishes a working relationship.				
10. Relates with physicians; establishes a working relationship.				
11. Relates with service supervisor and unit secretary; establishes a working relationship.				
12. Conducts self professionally; does not eat or smoke on the floor.				
13. Demonstrates a sensitivity to patient needs.				
14. Demonstrates organizational ability.				

ADDITIONAL COMMENTS:

Nursing supervisor____________________R.N.

Anecdotal records—L.P.N.; Nurses' aide (Att.)

Name____________________ Total of patients assigned__________

Date____________________ Functional assignment__________

	YES	NO	SOMETIMES	COMMENTS
Hygiene and physical comfort of patient				
1. Oral hygiene given appropriately.				
2. Bath given appropriately.				
3. Bed made appropriately.				
4. Skin care given.				
5. Hair groomed.				
6. Nails clean.				
7. Positioning comfortable and correct.				
Activity of patient				
1. Performed as indicated.				
Safety of patient				
1. Height of bed low.				
2. Side rails on bed of patient whose condition warrants.				
3. Patient's equipment kept within his reach.				
4. Call light in place.				
5. Environment safe and clean.				
a. Assigned rooms straightened.				
b. Equipment put back when use finished.				
Nutrition				
1. Patients assisted with food trays.				
2. Fluids given or restricted appropriately.				
Emotional needs of patients				
1. Each patient treated with respect and kindness.				
2. Listened to attentively.				
3. Kindness shown to family.				
Assigned procedures				
1. Vital signs taken correctly and on time.				
2. Specimens started and collected appropriately.				
3. Temperatures taken correctly and on time.				
4. Isolation technique carried out correctly.				
5. Enemas given correctly.				

	YES	NO	SOMETIMES	COMMENTS
Charting				
1. Vital signs charted correctly.				
2. T.P.R.s charted correctly.				
3. Admission note charted correctly.				
4. Intake and output charted correctly.				
5. L.P.N.'s observations pertinent and complete.				
Initiative				
1. Arrives on time for work.				
2. Answers lights promptly.				
3. Seeks to aid co-worker.				
4. Utilizes time well.				
5. Checks back on patients frequently.				
6. Makes pertinent contributions during conference.				
7. Reports immediately to team leader any change in patient's condition.				
Functional assignment				
1. Prepares patients for breakfast and lunch.				
2. Passes water.				
3. Maintains intern's laboratory.				
4. Maintains treatment room.				
5. Maintains kitchen.				
6. Sees that scale is in order.				

ADDITIONAL COMMENTS:

Signature________________________R.N.

Tape-recorded change-of-shift report

PURPOSE: To facilitate the fulfillment of the professional nurse's legal responsibility to communicate pertinent information necessary for continuity of patient care management.

DEFINITION: Report, given by the professional nurse at the end of each 8-hour shift, that involves the transfer of responsibility for patient care.

GENERAL INSTRUCTIONS:

Recording time: Approximately 45 minutes before beginning of following shift.

Receiving time: 7 A.M., 3 P.M., 11 P.M.

Place: As designated on each unit.

Recorders: Team leaders of offgoing shift.*

Receivers: Team leaders, clinical nurses, medication nurses, nurse clinicians, supervisors.

Clarification time: Approximately 5 minutes per team, during which the oncoming team leader may seek information not provided in the taped report and during which the offgoing team leader may provide any last-minute information.

PREPARATION FOR RECORDING REPORT:

1. Organize necessary information.
   a. Make recent nursing rounds.
   b. Take report from team members.
   c. Check for any new information regarding admissions, discharges, transfers, tests, medications, etc.
   d. Review Kardex.
2. Notify secretary and team members which team leaders will be recording first and second.

CONTENT OF REPORT:

1. State date, time, team, and recorder.
2. Identify each individual patient report with room and bed numbers, name, marital status (Mrs., Miss, Mr.), age.
3. Report only pertinent *new* or *changed* information regarding the following.
   a. Current condition.
   b. Symptoms.
   c. Therapeutic measures—treatments, diagnostic tests, medications, and surgery.
   d. Complications of any kind.
   e. Medical history.
   f. Basic needs—activity, hydration, elimination, nutrition, hygiene, and sensory stimulation.

*The recorder (offgoing team leader) may *not* leave the unit until after this report has been completed. The recorder retains full responsibility for the team until after this report has occurred.

g. Patient and/or family's reactions to illness and hospitalization.
h. Psychosocial background.
i. Discharge plans.

4. At conclusion of report you may include messages such as these: "all coumadin has been given" or "listen for message from unit manager, supervisor, or nurse clinician."

GENERAL INSTRUCTIONS FOR CARE OF MACHINE:

1. Be familiar with any literature provided with the tape recorder that includes information and directions for recording, playing, replacement of batteries, use of microphone, etc.
2. Microphone should be set on desk when recording—*not* held in hand.
3. To *record*
   a. Plug in microphone and have its switch in "off" position.
   b. Depress "Red Record" button and "Play-Rec" buttons simultaneously.
   c. Utilize microphone switch to control "off" and "on."
   d. If it is necessary to "rewind" or if any other buttons are depressed, *must* begin recording sequence from step "a."
   e. At end of report, rewind to the beginning for the receiver.
4. To *listen*
   a. Make sure the "Red Record" button is *not* depressed.
   b. Depress "Play-Rec" button only and push microphone switch to "on" position.
5. Precautions:
   a. *Never* leave machine plugged into electrical outlet when not in use.
   b. *Never* attempt to repair machine. Refer to unit manager.

Walking-planning rounds

DEFINITION: Nursing team (team leader and team members) visits each patient on the team in a systematic manner for the purpose of involving the patient in his plan of care, clarifying and revising the plan, and directing the personnel regarding specifics of the patient's care.

OBJECTIVES:

A. To involve patient in planning his care
   1. Team leader introduces herself and team member who will be giving care to the patient.
   2. Team leader updates care plan as she talks to and listens to patient.
   3. Patient can ask questions of the nurse concerning his care.
   4. Team leader teaches the patient concerning his care—explains n.p.o., orders to restrict or force fluids, save urine, x-ray procedures, etc.
   5. Team leader and team member can handle patient's needs at the time of making rounds—place on bedpan, roll head of bed up and down, give drink of water, hang intravenous fluids, etc.

B. To provide an opportunity for personnel teaching
   1. Team leader can give specific directions to the nursing personnel regard-

ing patient treatments such as decubitus care, bladder irrigation, spot checks, and dressings.
2. Since "one picture is worth a thousand words," this provides for a more thorough and accurate clarification report.

C. To provide an opportunity to assess patient's environment
1. Team leader can direct nursing personnel to clean bedside stands, overbed tables, discontinue monitor, discontinue ice mattress, etc.
2. Team leader can direct nursing and housekeeping personnel to keep hall clean and uncluttered.

D. To provide for better utilization of time and nursing personnel
1. Multiple teams can have report at the same time.
2. Patients' lights are constantly visible, since personnel are out in the halls.
3. Team leader is available when physicians come to ask questions and in turn team leader can ask physician questions.
4. Press team leader to set up medications earlier and/or make rounds with physicians.
5. Scheduled for approximately 7:30 A.M. and/or 3:30 P.M. Can begin earlier if team members and team leader are ready.
6. Duration is about 20 to 30 minutes.

Daily census

CONTENT

1. Nursing station—In this space identify the floor or special area that the census sheet will include.
2. Date—Specify day that the census will cover.
3. Room and bed number—List the rooms and beds in numerical order in this column. The bed numbering system should be as follows.
   a. For semiprivate rooms, face the beds and assign number 1 to the bed on the far right. Continue numbering sequentially, moving to the left.
   b. Designate sun porch beds as SP, followed by the bed number, and hall beds as H, followed by the bed number. The bed number in these areas is determined in the same manner as room bed numbers.
4. Name—Write the name of the patient occupying that bed.

In the next column—labeled Service—classify the patient as to private or service. Use P for private and S for service.

5. Medical service—Indicate the service to which the patient is assigned—Medicine, Surgery, OB, etc.
6. Census statistics—All transfers, room changes, admissions, discharges, and deaths should be recorded in this column. On all transfers, the room number from which the patient came or to which he is going should be indicated immediately following the code that corresponds to the change.

7-11. Sections 7 through 11 are designated as follows: (7) Amb. (ambulation and movement), (8) Feed (feedings), (9) Bath (bathing), (10) Cont. (continence), and (11) Special duty. These are the five major functions of dependency on the nursing staff. Four of the five functions are further evaluated by the degree of dependence and required patient care and are categorized as follows: Self (self-care), Partial (partial care), and Total care. The fifth function is Special duty, which pertains to special nursing care attention. A detailed list of terms and description of the patient typing system is included in this discussion. Each patient is to be typed separately, by measuring each of the five functions and determining what category best describes the patient. The number under the appropriate category is then circled.

12. Total points—This is the total point accumulation for each patient when the circled numbers are added across the page and entered in the column.
13. Patient type—The patient type is determined by the total points accumulated. The total points are compared to the point range listed here, to identify the patient type. The appropriate number showing the patient type will be entered in the patient type column.
14. Patient condition—This column is to show the patient's condition as determined by night charge nurse, using the following categories: good, fair, serious, and critical.

Census statistics—The listing of codes to be entered in column (6) describing the movement of patients.

A—Admission	TI —Transfer in
D—Discharge	TO—Transfer out
RC—Room change	DH—Death

Patient type—The listing or range of points to be used in determining the patient type.

0-1 point —Type 1
2-3 points—Type 2
4-7 points—Type 3
8-10 points—Type 4
11-15 points—Type 5

An example of the daily census report is shown in Fig. 4.

Preparation

The responsibility for the daily preparation of the daily census report is divided between nursing service and patient services, each being responsible for a definite area, as follows.

Patient services

1. The patient services department representative at each nursing station (normally the unit secretary) will be responsible for seeing that the report is filled out with the following data: nursing station, date, room and bed number, patient's name, service, and census statistics. This data will be on the report before it is given to the team leader at 2 P.M. each day. After the team leader (or charge nurse) has completed the evaluation and typing of patients,

DAILY CENSUS REPORT — 12:00 MIDNIGHT

NURSING STATION 3rd floor (1) — DATE May 1, 1973 (2)

(3) Room AND BED NO.	(4) PATIENT NAME	SERVICE	(5) MED SERV	(6) CENS STAT	(7) AMB & M 0-Self Care 1-PART Care 2-Tot. Care	(8) FEED 0-Self Care 2-Part Care 3-Tot. Care	(9) BATH 0-Self Care 2-Part Care 3-Tot. Care	(10) CONT 0-Self Care 2-Part Care 3-Tot. Care	(11) SP DUTY 3 PTS.	(12) TOT. PNTS.	(13) PT. TYPE	(14) PT. COND
302^1	mrs A				1	2	2	3	3	11	5	F
302^2	mrs. B				2	0	2	2	3	9	4	F
303^1	mrs. C				2	2	2	2	3	11	5	G
303^2	miss D				1	1	2	2	3	9	4	S
304^1	mrs E				2	2	2	2	0	8	4	S
304^2	mrs F				0	0	2	2	0	4	3	F
308^1	mrs G				0	0	0	0	3	3	2	F
308^2	miss H				2	2	2	2	0	8	4	F
309^1	mrs I				0	0	0	0	3	3	2	F
309^2	mrs J				2	3	3	3	3	14	5	S
310	mrs. K				2	3	3	3	3	14	5	S
314	miss L				0	0	2	2	3	7	3	S
317	mrs M				2	2	2	2	3	11	5	S
318^1	mrs N				0	0	0	0	3	3	2	G
318^2	miss O				1	2	2	2	0	7	3	F
321	mrs P				0	0	0	0	3	3	2	F
322	mrs Q				2	2	2	2	3	11	5	F
334^1	mrs R				2	3	3	3	3	14	5	C
334^2	mrs S				2	3	3	3	3	14	5	C
338^1	mrs T				2	3	3	3	3	14	5	C
338^2	mrs U				0	0	0	0	0	0	1	G
	Work units		Category		I =	1						
					2 =	8						
					3 =	9						
					4 =	16						
					5 =	45						
			Total			79 ÷ 14 = 5.6 or 6 people for direct pt care.						

CENSUS STATISTICS
A--Admitted
D--Discharge
RC-Room Change & Room No.
TI-Trans. In & Room No.
TO-Trans. Out & Room No.
DH-Death

PATIENT TYPE Points	Type
0-1	Type 1
2-3	Type 2
4-7	Type 3
8-10	Type 4
11-15	Type 5

PATIENT CONDITION
Good
Fair
Serious
Critical

STAFFING Skill	AM	PM	EVE
RN	2	2	1
LPN	4	2	2
T.A. & Other	2	2	1
Unit Sec.	1	1	
Unit Supr	1/2		

CENSUS BY SERVICE	MED	NEUR	PSY	DERM	SURG GEN	PL SURG	ENT	OPTH	GU	ORTH	GYN	OB	NEW BORN	TOT
Last Report														
Admitted (+)														
Transfers In (+)														
Discharges (−)														
Transfers Out (−)														
Deaths (−)														
12:00 Census														

Fig. 4. (Modified from Carter, Joan, et al.: Standards of nursing care, New York, 1972, Springer Publishing Co., Inc.)

she will return the report to the unit secretary for adding point totals and recording the patient type on the form.

2. The night unit secretary (also the day unit secretary) will make any necessary changes in the report and note any changes to the team leader or charge nurse.
3. The census by service section of the report will be filled in by the night unit secretary.
4. It is also the responsibility of the unit manager to confirm that the unit secre-

tary is filling out the report correctly and to fill in the staffing information required.

Nursing service

1. Team leader (or charge nurse in the team leader's absence) will evaluate each patient at the nursing area. This will be done at 2 P.M. each day. The nurse in charge at night will make any necessary changes in he report caused by admissions, discharges, etc.
2. The night charge nurse will be responsible for filling in the patient condition information section.
3. The night supervisor should review the report for completeness and accuracy and deliver it to the admitting office by 2 A.M.

DISTRIBUTION

The report will be filled out in duplicate at the nursing station.

The original copy will be delivered to the admitting office where three duplicated copies will be made and distributed in the following manner:

ORIGINAL	To the accounting office
COPY 1	To be retained in the admitting department for statistical information
COPY 2	To the information desk or switchboard for patient condition information
COPY 3	To the director of nursing service for staffing information

The carbon copy of the original is to be retained at the nursing station. This copy need be kept only until the next day's census report is completed.

DAILY TIMETABLE FOR PATIENT CATEGORIZATION AND CENSUS

11:00 A.M.-2:00 P.M.: Unit secretaries will list all patients who have been or are presently on their floor. Patients who have been on the floor but are no longer there will be recorded on the sheet and their movements indicated by discharge, transfer, room change, etc. The unit secretary will give the census sheet to the team leader promptly at 2 P.M.

2:00 P.M.-3:30 P.M.: The team leader will type each patient on the floor according to the amount of nursing care required in the five categories listed on the census sheet. The nurse will give the census sheet back to the unit secretary before leaving.

3:30 P.M.-11:00 P.M.: The unit secretary will total up the points for each patient and type that patient in accordance with the total points. All admissions, discharges, and transfers during that time period will be recorded on the census sheet. The census by service for that floor should be completed at 11 P.M. This information should be double checked for accuracy. At 11 P.M. the unit secretary should give the census sheet to the charge nurse.

11:00-11:30 P.M.: The charge nurse will assess the patient's condition (good, fair, serious, or critical) and record the condition. Also, she should type any patients who have been admitted since 2 P.M. on the census sheet. She should then give the form back to the unit secretary.

11:30 P.M.: The census sheet should be complete at this time. The unit secretary should check the sheet for completeness; if it is not complete, she is responsible for adding the missing information.

11:30 P.M.-12:00 midnight: All room changes, transfers, admissions, and discharges will be properly recorded and the necessary information added to the sheet.

2:00 A.M.: The census sheet on each floor and/or unit will be picked up by the night supervisor and delivered to the admitting office.

Patient typing system

The following patient typing system categorizes patients in terms of the five major functions of dependency on the nursing staff and the three categories of patient care listed.

Functions of dependency

1. Ambulation
2. Feeding
3. Bathing
4. Continence
5. Special duty (postoperative care, oxygen, isolation, any unusual care, or doctor's orders)

Categories of patient care

1. Self-care
2. Partial care (nurse assistance)
3. Total care

The assigning of a point system to the functions of dependency, coupled with the category of patient care required, establishes the patient typing.

Classifications used in various hospital areas are indicated in the accompanying lists.

Medical and surgical areas

(Not including ICU, CVR, CCU, psychiatric area, obstetrics area, or nursery)

Functions of dependency	*Points*		
	Self-care	*Partial care*	*Total care*
Ambulation	0	1	2
Feeding	0	2	3
Bathing	0	2	3
Continence	0	2	3
Special duty	0	0	3

Type 1 patient— 0- 1 point
Type 2 patient— 2- 3 points
Type 3 patient— 4- 7 points
Type 4 patient— 8-10 points
Type 5 patient—11-15 points

Obstetrics area

Functions of dependency	*Points*		
	Self-care	*Partial care*	*Total care*
Feeding	0	2	3
Bathing	0	2	3
Continence	0	2	3
First-day care, special duty	0	3	3
Cesarean section care, first-day only	0	3	3

Type 1 patient— 0- 1 point
Type 2 patient— 2- 3 points
Type 3 patient— 4- 7 points
Type 4 patient— 8-10 points
Type 5 patient—11-15 points

Nursery

Type 1 patient—Normal care.
Type 2 patient—Special care (premature infant, infant with birth defects, etc.).

Special care nursing areas
(ICU, CCU, CVR, any intensive care sections)

All patients in the special care nursing areas would normally be in a condition of total dependence. The types are then classified as follows:

Type 1 patient—Close supervision (including IVs, medications, dressing, etc.) and monitoring.
Type 2 patient—Type 1 plus moderate special procedures (tracheotomy, etc.).
Type 3 patient—Type 2 plus intensive special procedures (24-hour care).

Psychiatric area

Type 1 patient—Patient requiring minimal nursing care and independent in daily activities; may require occasional counseling.
Type 2 patient—Patient who requires a moderate amount of nursing care and can accomplish daily activities with minimal instruction and observation.
Type 3 patient—Patient who requires some intensive nursing care and whose activities must be partially controlled with periodic treatment, observation, and/or instruction.
Type 4 patient—Patient who requires intensive nursing care and whose activities must be rigidly controlled with continuous treatment, observation, and/or instruction.

Definition of terms

Ambulation and movement

Self-care: Patient can get in and out of bed without assistance.

Partial care: Patient needs one person to assist him in getting in and out of bed. He may need someone to help him walk.

Total care: Patient needs two or more persons to assist him in and out of bed. He may need two persons to help him walk or two or more persons to lift him from bed to cart. He may need to be turned and given passive exercise.

Feeding

Self-care: Patient can cut his own food, feed himself, and brush his own teeth.

Partial care: Patient needs help with preparing his food and brushing his teeth.

Total care: Patient must be fed, requires intravenous therapy, or tube feedings.

Bathing

Self-care: Patient can completely bathe himself.

Partial care: Patient requires assistance with his bath.

Total care: Patient needs to be given a complete bath.

Continence

Self-care: Patient goes to bathroom by himself.

Partial care: Patient needs assistance in getting to bathroom or needs to be offered the bedpan or urinal. Patient needs to be handed washcloth.

Total care: Patient is incontinent, involuntary, has an indwelling catheter, or has external urinary drainage.

Special duty—for patient who needs:

Isolation technique.

Turning, coughing, and deep breathing (more frequently than every 2 to 3 hours).

Extensive decubitus care or special dressings such as burn dressings.

Vital signs more frequently than every 4 hours.

Close observation of general condition, as needed by (1) unconscious, confused, or senile patient or (2) patient with a condition that may change quickly—a patient with head injuries, a patient with acidosis or alkalosis, etc.

Monitors.

Tracheostomy care and/or suctioning.

Respirators (only if the nurse is responsible for administration).

Drainage tubes (chest bottles; Hemovacs; gastrointestinal devices (nasal-gastric tubes, gastrostomy tubes, sump tubes, ureteral catheters, etc.)

Oxygen therapy (only if the nurse is responsible for administration).

Traction devices.

Stryker frames.

Radium precautions.

Colostomy and/or ileostomy care.

Continuous bladder irrigation.

Therapy for hemorrhage.

Criteria for staffing

Many variables affect the staffing of nursing units. However, there are methods that provide factual information for determining the total number and kinds of staff required.*

In one group of hospitals using the criteria for staffing described by Carter and co-workers, it has been found that one R.N., L.P.N., or nurses' aide can give direct patient care (bathing, feeding, etc.) to a number of patients equal to a total of 14 to 15 work units.

One professional nurse can supervise the physical and task-oriented care given by the nonprofessional staff and can give the professional care necessary (assessment, planning, and evaluation of patient care, administration of medications, intravenous fluid administration, etc.) to a group of patients no larger than 16 to 18 and including no more than 2 or 3 type 5 patients. If there are more than 16 patients and the need for more professional care (type 5), then there must be more R.N.s accordingly.

The largest number of nursing staff should be on the 7 to 3 shift. Staffing is based on the work load of the 7 to 3 shift. This shift covers two feeding periods, the bathing, and the largest number of procedures and tests. The 3 to 11 shift should equal three fourths the number of staff on the 7 to 3 shift. The 11 to 7 shift requires one half as many as the day shift staffing pattern.

These criteria are based on the patient care needs of an acute hospital unit and are not applicable to a self-care unit.

Criteria for assigning patient care

PURPOSE: To define guidelines, which the team leader utilizes to determine and evaluate patient care assignments so that these will fulfill the specified standards for nursing care.

USE:

1. Patient classification system is used as a basis for the division of patient work load
   a. Complete and consider the census and condition sheet as summary of overall situation.
   b. The average amount of direct care corresponds with the patient classification. There are distinctions in the intermediate (between 2 and 3) and in the total (between 4 and 5) care; the higher the number of the patient type, the more complex the care.

Type 1 patient	Minimal care	= 1 work unit
Type 2 patient	Intermediate care	= 2 work units
Type 3 patient	Intermediate care	= 3 work units
Type 4 patient	Total care	= 4 work units
Type 5 patient	Total care	= 5 work units

*See Carter, Joan, et al.: Standards of nursing care: a guide for evaluation, New York, 1972, Springer Publishing Co., Inc.

c. The classification (type) thus determines the work units assigned. For example, a type 2 patient is 2 work units. If there are 10 type 2 patients, they represent 20 work units. A type 5 patient is 5 units of work. Four type 5 patients represent 20 units of work.

d. When the total work units have been computed, the number is divided by 14 to ascertain the number of staff required to give the physical care.

e. When all patient care has been allocated, no team member's assignment should total more than 14 to 15 units of work. This figure is based on maximum work load established by Connor at Johns Hopkins. This study was confirmed by an activities study conducted at Saint Louis University Hospitals (Carter et al.).

2. Adjustments are made (Fig. 5), considering the existing resources:
   a. Number of personnel available.
   b. Level of personnel (R.N., L.P.N., Att.).
   c. Educational preparation, abilities, and personality of each staff member.

NURSING ASSIGNMENT RECORD

DIVISION 8 NURSING SERVICE 7-3^{30} DATE May 2, 1973

NURSES	ON DUTY A.M.	ON DUTY P.M.	A.M. ASSIGNMENTS	P.M. ASSIGNMENTS	MEAL HOURS NOON	MEAL HOURS P.M.
					Coffee at 9	
Mary Jones Rn	✓		Team leader north		11^{30}	
Alice Brown Rn	✓		822¹ mr. Hall ⑤ 810 mr. Brown ⑤ 817 mr. Smith ⑤ (15)		C.B. 9^{15} 11^{00}	
Jane Hall L.P.n	✓		811 mr. Abel ④ 820 mr. Kline ④ 822² mr. Coy ④ 812 mr. Cahill ② (14)	all Vital signs 10 - 2	C.B. 9^{00} 11	
Mary Johnson LPn.	✓		802¹ mrs. McBride ④ 802² mrs. Hicks ④ 803¹ mrs Warren ④ 804¹ mrs Bell ② (14)	Take 7-11 Temperatures	C.B. 9^{15} 11^{30}	
Mrs Barr L.P.n	✓		805¹ mr. Robb ⑤ 805² mr. Hart ⑤ 806 mrs. Fox ⑤ (15)	Straighten utility Room	C.B. 9^{30} 12^{00}	
Mrs Jenkins NA			807 mr. Lamb ② 808¹ mr. Crim ② 809 mrs. Collins ② 813 mrs. Ball ② 814 mrs. McClain ② 816 mrs. Berry ② 818 mr. Roby ② (14)	Clean medicine Room	C.B. 9^{30} 12^{30}	
				Walking rounds 7^{30} a.m. Team Conference 1^{30} 805¹ mr. Robb		

Fig. 5

3. If the unit has patients who are all in the type 1 or type 2 classification and minimal professional care is required, one R.N. may be sufficient for the supervision of nonprofessional personnel caring for 60 to 80 patients. This again must be carefully assessed according to existing resources.

Activities list

Some employees find that they cannot accomplish their assigned work load in the allotted time. In a study completed here by Carter et al., to determine the average length of time required for the completion of the various activities by our own employees, the data we obtained, tabulated here, do not differ significantly from the findings of "CASH" of California.

If you have employees on your team who cannot complete their assignment in the allocated time, we suggest that you give them a copy of the activities list. Ask them to time themselves and bring their performance up to the standard length of time required for the various activities.

Code	*Activity*	*Level of competence*	*Standard (minutes)*
1	Admission of newborn	L.P.N., R.N.	30
2	Admission to postpartum	L.P.N., R.N.	10
3	Admit new patient	L.P.N., R.N.	20
4	Admit new patient, assessment by team leader	R.N.	35
5	Ambulate patients	Att., L.P.N., R.N.	30
6	Analyze oxygen concentration in nursery	L.P.N., R.N.	5
7	Answer call lights	Att., L.P.N., R.N.	5
8	Aqua K-pad	L.P.N., R.N.	20
9	Assist patient to sit up, back to bed, or up in chair	Att., L.P.N., R.N.	10
10	Assist with bedpan, urinal, or commode	Att., L.P.N., R.N.	10
11	Assist with circumcision	L.P.N., R.N.	15
12	Attend seminars and demonstrations	Att., L.P.N., R.N.	50
13	Backrub	Att., L.P.N., R.N.	8
14	Blanket technique in nursery	Att., L.P.N., R.N.	3
15	Bone marrow aspiration	L.P.N., R.N.	30
16	Bottle feeding of infant in nursery	Att., L.P.N., R.N.	20
17	Breast-feeding for infant	Att., L.P.N., R.N.	10
18	Cardiac arrest	R.N.	60
19	Catheter irrigation	L.P.N., R.N.	10
20	Catheterization	L.P.N., R.N.	20
21	Change catheter bags	Att., L.P.N., R.N.	10
22	Change dressings or reinforce	L.P.N., R.N.	10
23	Changing diaper	Att., L.P.N., R.N.	3
24	Charting	L.P.N., R.N.	2
25	Check medicine cards with Kardex	L.P.N., R.N.	15
26	Clarification report	R.N.	2
27	Clean catch specimen	Att., L.P.N., R.N.	10
28	Clean bassinet	Att., L.P.N., R.N.	15
29	Cleansing enema, prepackaged	Att., L.P.N., R.N.	30
30	Cleansing enema, soapsuds	Att., L.P.N., R.N.	30
31	Clinitest-Acetest	L.P.N., R.N.	10
32	Close charts	L.P.N., R.N.	2

Continued.

Code	*Activity*	*Level of competence*	*Standard (minutes)*
33	Collect intake and output records	Att., L.P.N., R.N.	5
34	Collect soiled linen from nursery	Att., L.P.N., R.N.	4
35	Collect specimen requested	Att., L.P.N., R.N.	5
36	Collect urine specimen from infant	Att., L.P.N., R.N.	10
37	Colostomy care	L.P.N., R.N.	30
38	Colostomy irrigation	L.P.N., R.N.	30
39	Complete bed bath	Att., L.P.N., R.N.	45
40	Complete checklist on pre-ops and chart	L.P.N., R.N.	10
41	Conduct change-of-shift report	L.P.N., R.N.	1-2 per patient
42	Count narcotics	L.P.N., R.N.	2
43	Death procedure, physical care	L.P.N., R.N.	30
44	Decubitus care	L.P.N., R.N.	20
45	Discharge of infant	Att., L.P.N., R.N.	30
46	Discharge of patient	L.P.N., R.N.	10
47	Douche	L.P.N., R.N.	20
48	Eye instillation	L.P.N., R.N.	5
49	Feed patient	Att., L.P.N., R.N.	28
50	Feed patient, assisting	Att., L.P.N., R.N.	30
51	Fill ice bags	Att., L.P.N., R.N.	10
52	Gastric tube irrigations	L.P.N., R.N.	10
53	Give information to visitors	Att., L.P.N., R.N.	5
54	Hand-scrubbing technique	Att., L.P.N., R.N.	5
55	Heat applications	L.P.N., R.N.	10
56	Indirect patient care (assisting with proctoscopic examination)	Att., L.P.N., R.N.	30
57	Infant gavage	L.P.N., R.N.	20
58	Infant lavage	L.P.N., R.N.	30
59	Infant suctioning	L.P.N., R.N.	3
60	Initiation of cardiac monitoring	R.N.	20
61	IV (add to)	R.N.	5
62	IV (discontinue)	L.P.N., R.N.	5
63	IV (set up)	R.N.	10
64	Kardex rounds with unit resident	R.N.	4 per patient
65	Lumbar puncture	L.P.N., R.N.	30
66	Make bed, patient in bed	Att., L.P.N., R.N.	10
67	Make bed, patient not in bed	Att., L.P.N., R.N.	5
68	Make out assignments	R.N.	6 per patient
69	Making of linen pack	Att., L.P.N., R.N.	5
70	Midnight census	L.P.N., R.N.	2
71	Moist heat application	L.P.N., R.N.	15
72	Morning bath in nursery	Att., L.P.N., R.N.	30
73	OB observational rounds	L.P.N., R.N.	3
74	Oral or nasal suction	L.P.N., R.N.	15
75	Patient bed bath	Att., L.P.N., R.N.	20
76	Pass medications, injections	L.P.N., R.N.	3 per patient
77	Pass water	Att., L.P.N., R.N.	3
78	Passive exercises	L.P.N., R.N.	10
79	Patient P.M. care	Att., L.P.N., R.N.	10
80	Patient rounds	R.N.	2
81	Pelvic exam, Pap smear	L.P.N., R.N.	20
82	Perineal care	L.P.N., R.N.	10
83	PKU	L.P.N., R.N.	3
84	Posey restraint on bed patient	L.P.N., R.N.	20

Code	*Activity*	*Level of competence*	*Standard (minutes)*
85	Prepare patient for surgery or diagnostic procedure	L.P.N., R.N.	15
86	p.r.n. mealtime assistance	Att., L.P.N., R.N.	5
87	p.r.n. medications, charting, narcotics, barbiturates, sedatives	L.P.N., R.N.	5
88	p.r.n. oxygen therapy, nasal cannula and mask	L.P.N., R.N.	10
89	Proper attire for isolation	L.P.N., R.N.	15
90	Receive report	Att., L.P.N., R.N.	1-2 per patient
91	Receiving newborn	Att., L.P.N., R.N.	15
92	Record verbal or phone orders	R.N.	2
93	Removal of Foley catheter	L.P.N., R.N.	10
94	Removal of Levin or gastric tube	L.P.N., R.N.	10
95	Remove bedpan, urinal, or commode	Att., L.P.N., R.N.	5
96	Remove specimen container from isolation	Att., L.P.N., R.N.	15
97	Reposition patient	Att., L.P.N., R.N.	5
98	Restrain patient in chair	L.P.N., R.N.	20
99	Rounds with doctors	R.N.	2
100	Set up medications and chart	L.P.N., R.N.	2 per patient
101	Setting up room for isolation of patient	Att., L.P.N., R.N.	30
102	Shaving patient	Att., L.P.N., R.N.	30
103	Showing of babies	Att., L.P.N., R.N.	5
104	Sitz bath	Att., L.P.N., R.N.	30
105	Stryker frame	L.P.N., R.N.	20
106	Suppositories	L.P.N., R.N.	5
107	Taking fetal heart tone	L.P.N., R.N.	5
108	Taking infant to mother for the first time	L.P.N., R.N.	10
109	Team conference	R.N.	2
110	To remove infant from blanket in nursery	Att., L.P.N., R.N.	3
111	T.P.R. (oral or rectal)	Att., L.P.N., R.N.	2
112	Tracheostomy care	L.P.N., R.N.	15
113	Tracheostomy suctioning	L.P.N., R.N.	10
114	Transfer of patient	L.P.N., R.N.	2
115	Tube feedings, drip method	L.P.N., R.N.	20
116	Unsolicited visits to patient	Att., L.P.N., R.N.	2
117	Venous pressure	R.N.	10
118	Vital signs	Att., L.P.N., R.N.	3
119	Weigh patient, bed patient	Att., L.P.N., R.N.	10
120	Weigh patient, up patient	Att., L.P.N., R.N.	5
121	Weighing an infant	Att., L.P.N., R.N.	5

RECORDS AND NURSING ACTIVITIES

Additional materials concerning procedures and records for which the nursing staff has responsibility—largely selected from the preceding activities list—will complete this chapter. These again are presented in a form designed to facilitate independent study and self-directed learning.

Admission of the patient

PURPOSES:

To welcome the patient and family.

To orient the patient and family to the hospital environment.

To assess the immediate physical, psychosocial, and spiritual needs of the patient and family.

EQUIPMENT:

Charting forms

Admission nursing record.

Temperature record.

Blood pressure record.

Sphygmomanometer and stethoscope.

IVAC thermometer.

Scale.

Urine specimen container and label.

Patient "utility pack."

Gown, towel, and washcloth.

PROCEDURE:

1. Introduce the patient to any roommate and any personnel in the room.
2. Acquaint with and orient to the hospital regarding the following:
   a. Use of the call light and overbed table.
   b. Location of bathroom, bathtub, shower, clothes locker, and phones.
   c. Mealtimes.
   d. Chaplain's visit.
   e. Location and hours of cafeteria.
   f. Location of visitors' bathrooms.
   g. Visiting hours.
   h. Location of chapel.
3. Assist with unpacking and undressing if necessary.
4. Provide a "utility pack." Mark all items with the patient's first and last names. Use a "Magic Marker."
5. Supply a towel, washcloth, and gown.
6. Explain the routine admission urine.
7. Provide water per order of the physician or team leader.
8. Complete the admission section of the nursing record (T.P.R., B.P., etc.).
9. Report to the team leader and give her the admission note.

GUIDELINES FOR THE PROFESSIONAL ADMISSION ASSESSMENT: (Patient must be seen by the R.N. within 1 hour of arrival on the unit.)

1. Review information recorded in the admission note and information supplied by the person initiating the admission.
2. Review any history the patient has brought from physician.
3. Check the admitting diagnosis.
4. Interview the patient and/or family.
   a. Make sure that the patient has been introduced to the appropriate people and oriented to the hospital surroundings.
   b. Complete the section of the admission form related to drugs, etc.
   c. Briefly explain what "team leader" means.

   d. Supply information related to tests, diet, etc., if known.
   e. Utilize nursing history form as a guideline for obtaining information for initial assessment.
5. Observe and chart the following kinds of information:
   a. Reason patient states for being admitted (place in quotation marks)—Example: "high blood pressure."
   b. Reaction to hospitalization.
   c. Any history of the illness as described by the patient and/or family.
   d. Understanding of illness.
   e. Physical "handicaps"—Examples: deafness, blindness, paralysis, numbness.
   f. Pertinent information obtained through use of the nursing history form.
   g. Physical appearance, on observation—Examples: skin condition, position of extremities, pupils, level of consciousness, rash, cyanosis, contractures, shortness of breath.
   h. Emotional status—Example: appears upset, crying, apprehensive.
6. Answer any questions the patient and/or family may have.
7. If the patient still has valuables with him, advise that they be sent home or notify the unit manager, the admitting office, or the nursing supervisor (in that order).
8. If the patient is seriously ill, have the unit secretary notify the chaplain and the nursing supervisor.
9. If nursing care problems are anticipated, notify the nurse clinician.
10. The nurse must notify the physician. She may ask the unit secretary to call the doctor, but she must talk to him when he answers. If the doctor does not answer within 45 minutes to an hour, the nurse must call the private physician, give him the condition and ask if there are any orders that should be started before the house staff is located.
11. If the patient is a neurosurgical patient, his name and that of his physician will be written on a tape and placed at the entrance of the room by the unit manager.
12. The dietary department will automatically send a soft diet to the hall for the new admissions. If the patient is found to require n.p.o., the dietary department should be notified.
13. Explain visiting hours to relatives before they leave.
14. If the patient is to have surgery, obtain an operative permit before the relatives depart.

Nursing assessment follows.

NURSING ASSESSMENT INTERVIEW—HISTORY AND GUIDELINES FOR DATA BASE

The professional nurse must visit all new admissions within 1 hour after admission, or immediately if the patient's condition warrants. The information is used for preparing the nursing care plan.

General information

Reason for admission ____________________

Physical disability ____________________

How long have you been ill? ____________________

Family, home, and environment

Family ____________________

Who does cooking, shopping? ____________________

Who took care of you before admission ____________________

Personal habits

Sleep pattern ____________________

Elimination ____________________

Daily activities ____________________

Foods you do not like ____________________

Foods that disagree with you ____________________

Physical

General appearance ____________________

Acute, physical, or emotional state? ____________________

Family concern ____________________

Hearing ____________________

Communication problem ____________________

Personal belongings

Valuables safeguarded ____________________

Clothing secured ____________________

Nursing assessment

____

____

____

____

____

____

Nursing progress notes (Fig. 6)

PURPOSE: To provide a means of communicating and recording pertinent information concerning patient care.

PROCEDURE:

A. Admission section
   1. Completed by an R.N., L.P.N., or N.A.
   2. *All* items must be completed as follows:
      Date: Include month, day and year (example, 1/20/73).
      Time: Specify hour and encircle A.M. or P.M.
      Mode: X appropriate square.
      Age: As stated by patient or family member.
      Religion: As stated by patient or family member.
      Vital signs:
         Temperature: Specify whether rectal (R), by mouth (O), or axillary (A).
         Weight: Specify whether it is given in pounds (lb.) or in kilograms (kg.).
      Dentures, eyeglasses, contact lenses, or hearing aid: X appropriate square.
      Signature: Give first initial, last name, and status (R.N., L.P.N., or N.A.) of person completing this section.
   3. Person completing this section must
      a. Chart T., P., R., and weight on the T.P.R. graphic record.
      b. Chart B.P., P., and R. on the B.P. graphic record.

B. Professional admission assessment section
   1. Must be completed by an R.N. within *one* hour of patient's arrival on the unit.
   2. *All* items must be completed, as follows:
      Medications: X "none" or list names and/or prescription numbers of *all* medications the patient has been taking at home.
      Disposition: X appropriate square to indicate what was done with the patient's home medications.
      Allergies: Write "none known" or list *all* known or questionable drug or food sensitivities as stated by the patient or family member.
      Deformities, etc.: Describe in accurate and complete detail.
      Preadmission diet: List any special diet followed by the patient prior to admission.
      Orientation to unit: X appropriate square.
      House staff notified: Unit secretary or other person responsible specifices the hour and encircles A.M. or P.M.
   3. The R.N. then describes in detail all pertinent observations, interventions, and information gathered from the patient and/or family during the admission interview. This is written on the lined section of the nursing record. (A nursing history form may be used to aid in this assessment.) This note must be dated, timed, and signed. The professional nursing assessment summary should include

NURSING PROGRESS NOTES

Admission

DATE: 5/4/73 MODE: [ ] AMBULATORY [X] WHEELCHAIR [ ] STRETCHER AGE: 76

TIME: 2 ~~a.m.~~ p.m. RELIGION: Baptist

VITAL SIGNS: T 98° P 84 R 32 BP 124/70 HT 5'8" WT 44 kg

DENTURES: [ ] No [X] Yes — [X] upper [X] full [ ] partial; [X] lower [X] full [ ] partial

EYEGLASSES: [ ] No [X] Yes

CONTACT LENSES: [X] No [ ] Yes

HEARING AID: [X] No [ ] Yes

Signature: M. Jenkins NA

PROFESSIONAL ADMISSION ASSESSMENT

MEDICATIONS: None List Digitoxin 0.1mg 20 tab.
ORINASE 0.5 gm 6 tab.

Disposition: [ ] Kept [ ] Sent Home [ ] Med. Room [ ] At. Home

ALLERGIES and DRUG SENSITIVITIES: None

Deformities, bruises, prosthesis, open wounds, or scars: multiple marks on legs and arms

Preadmission diet: 1200 Cal. Orientation to Unit: [ ] Yes [ ] No

House Staff Notified: 2:10 ~~a.m.~~ p.m.

DATE	TIME	
5/4/73	2pm	Patient was admitted by wheelchair.
		Oriented as to time and place. She
		needed assistance in getting in bed.

Fig. 6

a. Patient's stated reason for admission.
b. Physical appearance.
c. Physical handicaps.
d. Names of medications patient has been taking or reasons for them if names are not known.
e. History and understanding of illness.
f. Reaction to illness and hospitalization.

NURSING PROGRESS NOTES
continued

Date	Time	
5/4/73	2 pm.	Patient states she has been ill for
		two weeks. She has a poor appo lite
		and has lost fifteen pounds. Daughter
		states she cannot get patient to eat.
		The patient has been Self-Sufficient until
		four days ago. She is now short of
		breath, pale, lips are Cyanotic, respirtions
		are shallow and rapid, Oxygen by Cannula
		Started. Housestaff notified. Chaplain notified.

Fig. 6, cont'd

g. Pertinent information on activities of home care and personal care.
h. Nursing actions taken.

4. If unable to obtain information on an admission item, write next to the item "not available" or "unobtainable."

C. Lined section
  1. Following the R.N.'s admission assessment, *only* an R.N. or an L.P.N. may chart in this section.

2. All entries must be dated and timed; indicate the day and month under the column marked "date" and indicate specific hour (example, 7^A, 9^P) under column marked "time."
3. *All* entries must be signed; use first initial, last name, and status (R.N., L.P.N.).
4. Discharge note must be written on every patient and must include the mode of transportation, who accompanied the patient, any medications sent home with the patient, and any other pertinent information.

Charting

PURPOSE: To provide a complete and accurate summary of the patient condition, activities, and progress.

POINTS OF EMPHASIS:

1. All notations must be made in *black ink.*
2. All *chart forms* must be identified by stamping or writing the patient's full name and room and bed number on the form before inserting in the chart.
3. No *erasures* may be made.
4. Any *error* must be neatly lined through and "error" written over it.
5. All *writing* must be neat and legible. Print, if writing is difficult to read.
6. All *signatures* must include first initial, last name, and title.
7. All *dates* must include month, day, and year.
8. All *times* must include the specific hour and have A.M. or P.M. designated.
9. Each shift must chart on every patient.

Use of the nursing care plan (Kardex)

PURPOSE:

1. To provide a comprehensive plan of the patient's medical and nursing care.
2. To provide a means of communication.

PRECAUTIONS AND POINTS OF EMPHASIS:

1. All notations should be printed, using pencil.
2. Red pencil should be used to note times of medications and treatments to be given between 11 P.M. and 7 A.M.
3. If the card is filled, a new card will be started and the old card filed on the unit for 3 months.
4. All nursing personnel are responsible for helping to keep the cards complete and current. Team leaders and ward clerks will be doing most of the writing, with the professional nurse and the service supervisor sharing responsibility.
5. Specific times should be written whenever possible (e.g., q. 2 hours—2^A, 4^A, 6^A, etc.).

EQUIPMENT:

Black pencil.
Red pencil.
Kardex card.
Blue pre-op. card.

Yellow, white, and pink medicine cards.

3 × 5 IV cards.

PROCEDURE:

A. Profile section

1. All information should be filled in at time of admission.
2. Information should be noted as follows:
    a. Date and time of admission to hospital.
    b. Height, weight, blood pressure, age on admission.
    c. Religion—note specific denomination.
    d. Fully attended—leave blank; chaplain will complete.
    e. O.R. procedure—note specific procedure and date.
    f. Room number—use room number plus a dash and then bed number (example, 803–1).
    g. Name—print last name in the lower part of designated area; indicate title and first name above.
    h. Diagnosis.
        (1) Keep current.
        (2) List primary diagnosis and any pertinent diagnoses.
    i. Service—use acceptable abbreviations (example, GU., MED., OB.).
    j. Physician—first initial and last name of private doctor; if no private doctor, print "service."

B. Drug section

1. Routine medicines.
    a. Print drug, dose, and route of administration; acceptable abbreviations may be used.
    b. Times per day—use abbreviations.
    c. Hours—use times designated by the hospital practice (night hours to be in red). A small a or p *must* follow designated time if the drug is to be given only once per day.
    d. Date started.
    e. Date discontinued.
        (1) To be noted for narcotics and drugs having specified time limits.
        (2) When drug is discontinued, cross through by using one line and insert date in the column.
    f. Daily h.s. medications.
    g. Anything ordered to be given more than one time must be so indicated.
2. p.r.n.
    a. Same as for a, d, and e listed for routine medicines.
    b. Sliding scale for insulin should be noted here.
3. Allergies—all *must* be noted in *red* pencil.

C. Record of tests and procedures

1. Date ordered and date scheduled should be noted. If unable to schedule, use date ordered and include explanatory note.

2. All one-time diagnostic tests or procedures that require special preparation.
3. All one-time urine or sputum specimens should be noted.
4. All one-time blood specimens requiring special preparation (e.g., 2-hour postprandial blood sugar, fasting blood sugar).
5. Name of any test, etc. requiring permit should be followed by a note saying either *Permit obtained* or *Permit not obtained.*
6. Cross through when test or procedure is completed.

D. Consultation section
1. Date, type, and/or person requested.

E. Daily or serial specimens and tests
1. Date ordered should be noted.
2. Daily tests requiring more than one specimen are noted. Examples: 7/10 24-hour sputum for AFB—start 7/11 7 A.M. end 7/12 7 A.M.; 7/10 sputum × 3—1, 2, 3.
3. If sliding scale is ordered, note should be written following double-voided specimen.

F. Nursing care section
1. Diet—date ordered and diet specified.
2. Nourishment—between-meal feedings noted and dated.
   a. Doctor's order.
   b. Nursing assessment.
   c. Times to be offered.
3. Feed—date assessed; use the terms *self, assist,* or *feed.*
4. Intake and output—date and indicate with check mark.
   a. Doctor's order.
   b. Nursing assessment.
   c. Use the words *limit* or *force* with amounts as indicated (write specific plan under interventions).
5. Bath—date assessed; use the terms *self, assist,* or *complete.*
6. Foley catheter.
   a. Date inserted and type.
   b. Catheter care—to be noted under intervention section.
7. Activity—if no doctor's order, nurse's assessment should be indicated.
   a. Date.
   b. If interval activity is indicated, specific time should be noted (e.g., t.i.d.—10, 2, 6, etc.).
8. Positioning—if no doctor's order, assess in relation to patient's condition.
   a. Date.
   b. The specific times for interval positioning (e.g., q. 2 hours—2, 4, 6, 8).
   c. Special devices and precautions may be noted in intervention section if room does not permit here.

9. Special skin or special mouth care.
   a. Doctor's order or nurse's assessment (e.g., q. 2 hours—2, 4, 6).
   b. Indicate special materials, frequency, date.
10. Weight—if no doctor's order, assess for need.
    a. Note interval for weighing (use specific dates).
    b. Time of day.
    c. Note type of scales.
11. Respiratory aids.
    a. Date.
    b. Type of therapy and intervals.
    c. Department responsible.
12. T.P.R.
    a. Date.
    b. Note specific times.
    c. Note rectal with (R).
    d. Note if apical pulses are to be taken.
    e. Checking pedal pulse is to be noted under intervention section.
13. Vital signs (this means blood pressure, pulse, respirations).
    a. Date.
    b. Specific times (even if routine).
    c. If indicated, note position of patient and which extremity.
14. Physical therapy, etc.
    a. Note type, intervals, and times.
    b. Note location of therapy (e.g., P.T. or patient's room).
    c. Department responsible.
15. Telephone numbers—list should include
    a. Numbers left by relatives not indicated on face sheet.
    b. Relationship of person.
16. Disposition of preadmission drugs—Examples: at bedside, returned to relatives, or in medicine room.
    a. If kept in medicine room, indicate ℞ number and amount of medication.
17. Clearly stated observations.
18. Date of assessments.
19. Clearly stated goals and interventions.
20. Initials of professional nurse.

G. Treatments section
   1. Date ordered.
   2. Type, duration, materials used.
   3. Hours specified.

H. Date of last B.M.

See Fig. 7 for an example of Kardex and Fig. 8 for examples of medicine tickets.

NURSING CARE PLAN

DIET: 5/24 Reg. Diet	NOURISHMENT: orange juice
FEED: assist	I & O: 5/24
BATH: assist	FOLEY: 5/26
ACTIVITY: 5/26 up in chair	A P 9-1-5 9
POSITIONING: Turn q 2 hrs (odd)	
SPECIAL SKIN CARE: Back Care am pm	
SPECIAL MOUTH CARE: 7 - 11 - 4	WEIGHT:
RESPIRATORY AIDS:	
TPR: 5/24 7-11-3 7-11-3	VITAL SIGNS: 5/24 7-11-3-7-11-3
PHYSICAL THERAPY AND OTHERS:	
TELEPHONE NUMBERS: Ted Brown 810 6428	
DISPOSITION OF PREADM. DRUGS: home with relative	

OBSERVATIONS	DATE: 5/24 GOALS & INTERVENTIONS
pale - chest	1. Prevent further Complications
pain (CA of	and maintain respiratory
Lung)	function.
	2. watch for chest pain,
	dyspnea, hemoptysis.
weak Cough	encourage to deep
	breath.
	Keep head of bed elevated.
poor appetite	allow family to
	bring in food she likes.
	give extra nourishment.
	Family does not want
	patient to know diagnosis.
	encourage family to let
	patient know.

Fig. 7

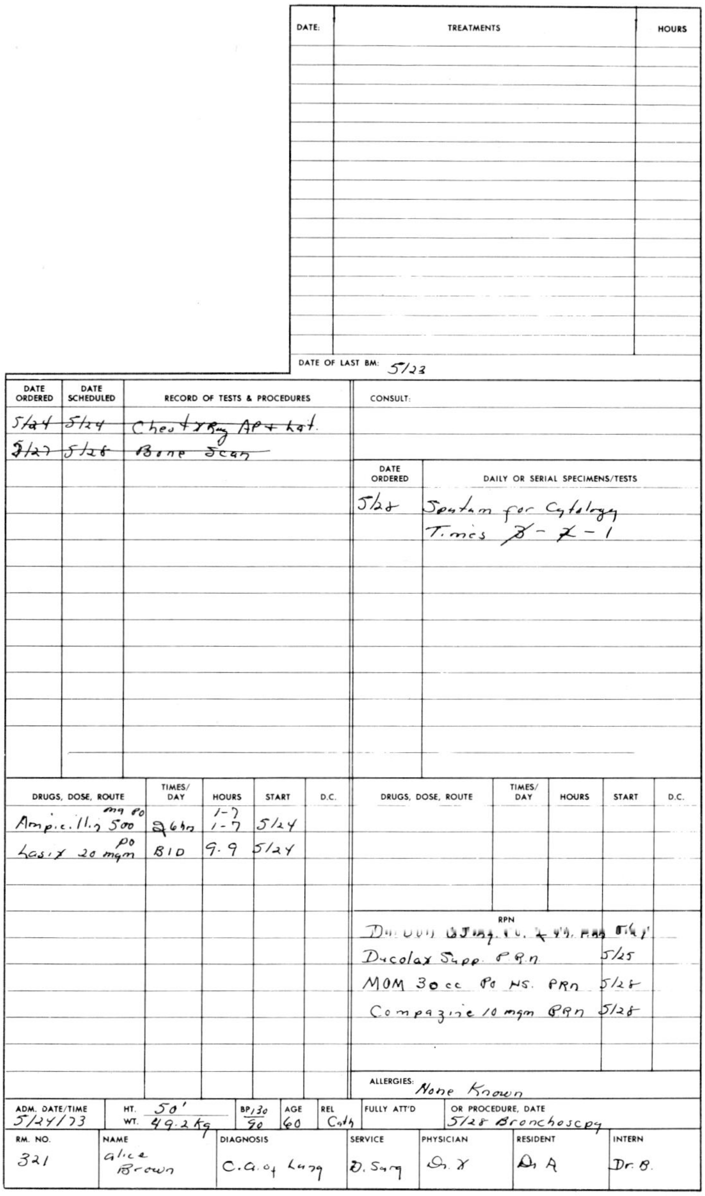

DATE:	TREATMENTS	HOURS

DATE OF LAST BM: 5/23

DATE ORDERED	DATE SCHEDULED	RECORD OF TESTS & PROCEDURES
~~5/24~~	~~5/24~~	~~Chest X Ray AP + Lat.~~
~~5/27~~	~~5/28~~	~~Bone Scan~~

CONSULT:

DATE ORDERED	DAILY OR SERIAL SPECIMENS/TESTS
5/28	Sputum for Cytology
	Times 3 - 2 - 1

DRUGS, DOSE, ROUTE	TIMES/ DAY	HOURS	START	D.C.
Ampicillin 500 mg po	q 6 hrs	1-7 1-7	5/24	
Lasix 20 mgm po	BID	9-9	5/24	

DRUGS, DOSE, ROUTE	TIMES/ DAY	HOURS	START	D.C.

RPN

[illegible]	
Ducolax Supp. P.R.N.	5/25
MOM 30 cc Po HS. PRN	5/28
Compazine 10 mgm PRN	5/28

ALLERGIES: None Known

ADM. DATE/TIME	HT. / WT.	BP	AGE	REL	FULLY ATT'D	OR PROCEDURE, DATE
5/24/73	HT. 50' WT. 49.2 Kg	130/90	60	Cath		5/28 Bronchoscpy

RM. NO.	NAME	DIAGNOSIS	SERVICE	PHYSICIAN	RESIDENT	INTERN
321	alice Brown	C.A. of Lung	D. Surg	Dr. X	Dr. A	Dr. B.

Fig. 7, cont'd

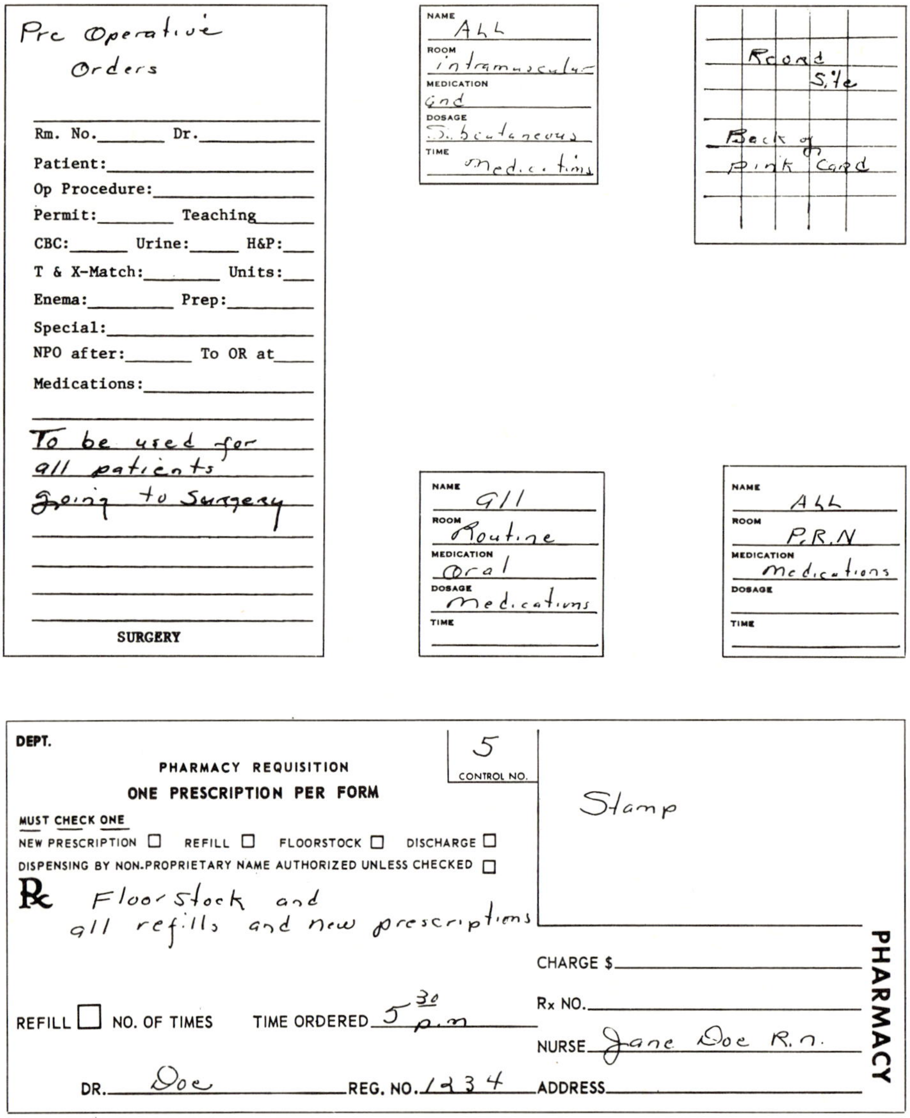
Pre Operative Orders

Rm. No.______ Dr.______
Patient:______
Op Procedure:______
Permit:______ Teaching______
CBC:______ Urine:______ H&P:______
T & X-Match:______ Units:______
Enema:______ Prep:______
Special:______
NPO after:______ To OR at______
Medications:______

To be used for all patients going to Surgery

SURGERY

NAME All
ROOM intramuscular
MEDICATION and
DOSAGE Subcutaneous
TIME medications

Record S/E
Back of pink Card

NAME all
ROOM Routine
MEDICATION Oral
DOSAGE medications
TIME

NAME ALL
ROOM P.R.N
MEDICATION medications
DOSAGE
TIME

DEPT.
PHARMACY REQUISITION
ONE PRESCRIPTION PER FORM
5 CONTROL NO.
Stamp
MUST CHECK ONE
NEW PRESCRIPTION ☐ REFILL ☐ FLOORSTOCK ☐ DISCHARGE ☐
DISPENSING BY NON-PROPRIETARY NAME AUTHORIZED UNLESS CHECKED ☐
℞ Floor stock and all refills and new prescriptions
CHARGE $______
Rx NO.______
REFILL ☐ NO. OF TIMES TIME ORDERED 5³⁰ p.m
NURSE Jane Doe R.N.
DR. Doe REG. NO. 1234 ADDRESS______
PHARMACY

Fig. 8

Care of patient with elastic stockings (antiembolic stockings)

PURPOSE: To improve venous circulation, which in turn both prevents and treats leg and foot edema and also helps prevent and treat thrombophlebitis and embolism.

POINTS OF EMPHASIS:

1. Physician will write order for antiembolic stockings, indicating whether he wants the stockings applied up to the knee or above the knee.
2. The professional nurse will measure the patient's legs to accurately fit the patient with the correct size stockings.

3. The patient's legs should be measured before he begins ambulating in the morning and while he is lying supine in bed. Use the measurements for the elastic stockings as directed in the manufacturer's literature.
4. On the treatment section of the Kardex should be written (a) apply the elastic stockings up to or above the knees, as ordered by the physician; (b) the times to remove the stockings; and (c) the amount of time the stockings should be left off.

PROCEDURE:

1. Elastic stockings are always removed for bathing; remove the stockings by starting at the top of the stockings and roll them down to the toes; do not attempt to pull the stockings off from the toes.
2. The stockings should be left off for at least 30 minutes in both the A.M. and the P.M.
3. Before reapplying the stockings the professional nurse or her designate should observe the patient's legs and feet for the following:
   a. Reddened areas.
   b. Size of legs and feet; note increase and/or decrease of edema.
4. Before reapplying the stockings, the professional nurse or her designate should dry the patient's legs and apply body powder to facilitate the reapplication of the stockings.
5. When reapplying the stockings, keep the following principles in mind:
   a. The stocking is applied to the entire foot and then advanced up the leg to below the knee or above the knee, as ordered by the physician; it should be rolled on evenly before the patient gets out of bed.
   b. The stockings should be smooth and snug.
   c. A stocking should not be so tight that it interferes with circulation.
6. Obtain a physician's order if he feels that the patient need not wear the stockings during the sleeping hours.
7. The professional nurse or her designate will chart in the nursing notes the time that the elastic stockings were taken off, the amount of time the stockings were left off, and any comments concerning the appearance of the patient's legs and feet; she should also note that the stockings were reapplied.

Care of patient with an arteriovenous (A-V) shunt (patient being hemodialyzed)

PURPOSE: To facilitate care of a patient's A-V shunt. This includes observing for signs of patency, preventing infection, and preventing hemorrhage.

PROCEDURE:

A. General care of patient on nursing division while not being dialyzed
   1. Weigh patient before and after dialysis on the same scale and chart on patient's T.P.R. graphic.
   2. Observe A-V shunt every 4 hours.
      a. Color—should be cherry red.
      b. Patency—listen with stethoscope over visible shunt for "swish" flow.

c. Temperature—shunt should feel warm.
d. Pulsation—place fingertips on shunt and feel pulse wave.

3. Take precautions to prevent clotting of shunt.
   a. No blood pressures are to be taken in the patient's arm having the A-V shunt.
   b. No tourniquets are to be applied to the arm with the shunt.
   c. No blood is to be drawn from the arm with the shunt.
4. Patient will be dialyzed 2 or 3 times a week, depending on his condition. The treatment will take place in the dialysis unit.
5. Diet—generally the patient will be receiving a diet consisting of the following:
   a. Restricted fluids (individualized according to patient need).
   b. Low potassium, low protein, and low sodium.
   c. Butter balls—if in acute renal failure.
6. Do not change dressing unless wet or soiled.
7. The two cannula clamps (bulldog clamps) *should* always be visibly clamped to the shunt dressing.

B. Care in event the shunt comes apart (patient will be hemorrhaging)
   1. Apply both clamps as quickly as possible—one to the arterial line and one to the venous line as close to the exit sites of shunt as possible. Make sure they are clamped securely.
   2. Clean both ends with alcohol, using sterile technique, and then connect the ends. The shunt connector must be in one of the two lines to reconnect the two lines.
   3. If the connector cannot be found, remember that a sterile connector is kept in the patient's medicine box on the nursing division. Sterile gloves must be used when replacing the connector. The hemodialysis nurse places this extra sterile connector in the patient's medicine box at the time the patient is admitted to the floor. When the patient is discharged, send the connector to the hemodialysis unit.
   4. Call the physician.

C. Care to be given if entire shunt comes out of patient's extremity
   1. Apply the blood pressure cuff over the A-V shunt site, since patient will be hemorrhaging. Pump cuff to 300 mm. Hg and deflate for 1 minute every 10 minutes.
   2. Call surgery resident who is caring for patient or the surgery resident on call, immediately; also call Dr. X, renal specialist.

D. Care of A-V shunt when dressing becomes *wet*
   1. Sterile technique is essential; sterile gloves must be worn; also a *mask* must be worn.
   2. Cleanse shunt site with povidone-iodine. Use one side of sterile 4 × 4 and then other side of the 4 × 4, making only one wipe with each side and wiping only away from the A-V site. Then discard the 4 × 4. Use one side of a 4 × 4 for each wipe of skin around the A-V shunt site.

3. Cleanse shunt site with alcohol after the povidone-iodine, using same procedure as for the cleansing with povidone-iodine.
4. Place one sterile 4 × 4 under shunt and one sterile 4 × 4 over shunt.
5. Wrap shunt with gauze dressing, which should be snug but not tight; be sure to expose tip of loop while wrapping; secure gauze with dressing tape.
6. If it is necessary to change the dressing, please call the hemodialysis nurse to check it. Do not hesitate to call the hemodialysis unit for assistance.

Blood pressure record (Fig. 9)

PURPOSE: To provide a continuous record of all blood pressures, pulses, respirations, central venous pressures, specific gravities, and temperatures.

PROCEDURE:

1. At midnight, draw a vertical line to divide the dates only.

   EXAMPLE:

DATE	1/20/74	1/21/74	1/22/74

   NOTE: Do *not* draw the vertical line to the bottom of the sheet.

2. Date: Write immediately after the vertical line. Include month, day, and year (example, 1/20/74).
3. Time: Write in the specific hour and indicate whether A.M. or P.M. (examples, 7^{A}, 11^{A}, 3^{P}).
4. Blood pressure reading:
   a. Chart beneath the correct time.
   b. Darken the appropriate dots for the systolic and diastolic pressures.
   c. Connect the dots: Systolic to systolic and diastolic to diastolic.
5. Pulse and respirations: Write vertically in the designated spaces beneath the correct B.P.

   EXAMPLE:

Pulse	108	84	92
Resp.	24	36	18

6. Blank spaces are provided at the bottom section of the sheet to chart the following:
   a. Central venous pressures (C.V.P.).
   b. Specific gravity of urine (Sp. Gr.).
   c. Elevated temperatures taken more frequently than every 4 hours.

USE: Write in the appropriate abbreviation and chart beneath the correct time at the top of the record.

C.V.P.	10	8	12	11
Sp. Gr.	1.010	1.010	1.010	1.010
Temp.	102^{2}	104	104^{2}	103^{6}

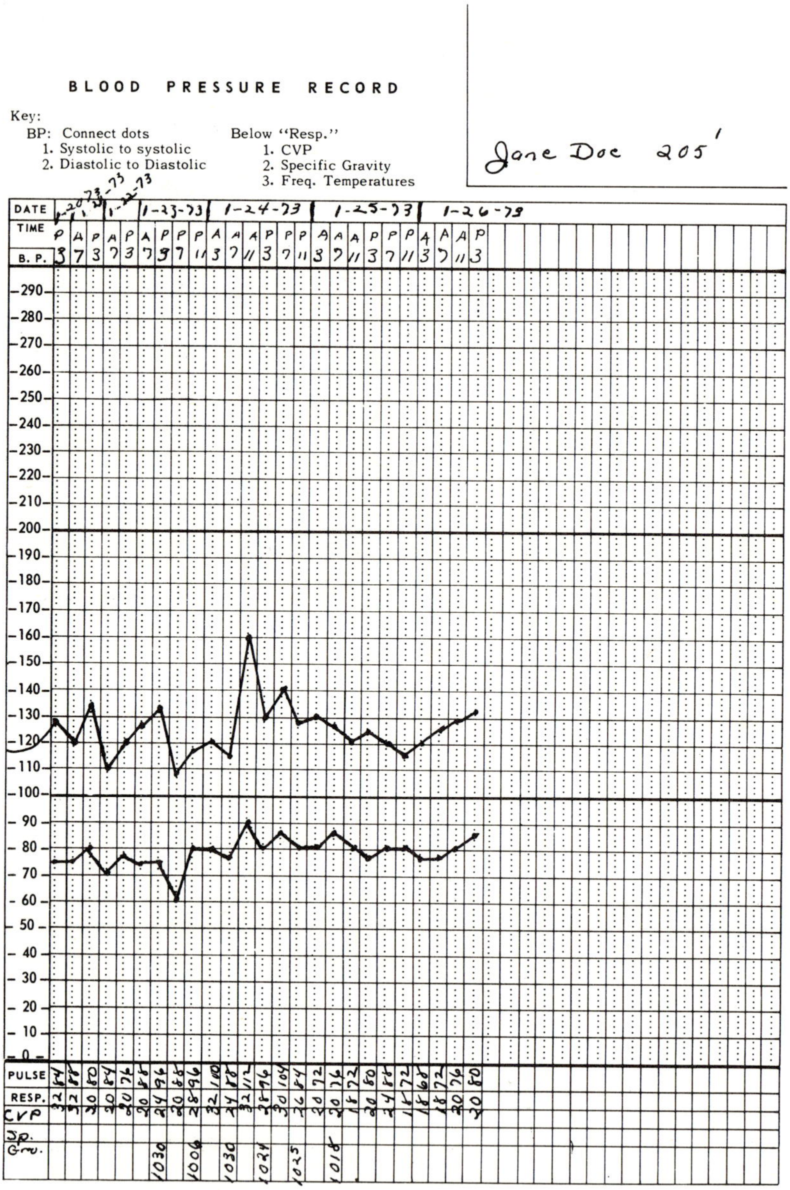

Fig. 9

Cardiac arrest procedure—step-by-step instructions

1. Make the diagnosis: Does cardiac arrest exist? Signs and symptoms are apnea, presence of carotid pulse, and dilation of pupils.
2. Obtain an airway: Extend the patient's head back as far as possible. Clear air passage of any obstruction and insert airway.
3. Call for help, from the room: Observe time and remember that you only have 4 minutes.

4. Prepare patient: Place the patient in a supine position on a firm surface; use the floor or lower the overbed table and place tray surface under patient.
5. Give a hard blow to chest. (This may restore the heartbeat.)
6. Begin ventilating patient.

   Mouth-to-mouth

   a. Remove any obstruction in throat or nasal passages.
   b. Tilt head all the way back and pull mandible forward.
   c. Keep victim's nostrils closed, using pressure of your fingers or cheek.
   d. Take deep breath, place wide-open mouth over victim's, and blow forcefully into the victim's mouth, making sure that his chest expands.
   e. Lift your head slightly and turn to observe chest action.
   f. Repeat at a rate of 10 to 15 times per minute.

   Mouth-to-nose

   a. Remove any obstruction in throat or nasal passages.
   b. Tilt victim's head all the way back and pull mandible forward.
   c. Keep his mouth tightly closed by pressure under the chin and lower lip.
   d. Take deep breath, place wide-open mouth over victim's nostrils, and blow into the victim's nose, making sure that his chest expands.
   e. Move your own head back and allow exhalation through the nostrils and open mouth.
   f. Repeat at a rate of 10 to 15 times per minute.
7. Begin external cardiac compression if there is no pulse.
   a. Place cardiac arrest board correctly under patient—must be on a hard surface.
   b. Place the heel of one hand over the lower half of the sternum and the heel of the other hand on top of the first.
   c. Keep the elbows straight and use the rocking motion of the body to depress the sternum 1½ to 2 inches.
   d. At the end of each stroke, the hands are relaxed to allow full chest expansion.
   e. Sternal compression is repeated once every second.

      NOTE: If alone —15 compressions, 3 breaths
      If 2 people— 5 compressions, 1 breath
8. Check the femoral or carotid pulse frequently to determine effective circulation.
9. Check the pupils for constriction.
10. When the arrest team arrives, the physician in charge assumes responsibility for the continuation of the procedure, and the nurses and unit manager present assume the following responsibilities:
    a. First-nurse responsibilities
       (1) Bring emergency cart to scene of arrest.
       (2) Obtain intubation equipment from first drawer—laryngoscope, endotracheal tube, guide wire, 10 ml. syringe, and clamp.
       (3) Break open medicine drawer.

Cardiac arrest record, including emergency drugs

NOTE:
1. Fill in time on top line.
2. Write dose under the time on the appropriate line.
3. Continue charting on other side.

Name ______________________

Room number ______________ Date ________

Time of episode ______________________

Time of expiration or arrest procedure ended ____________

Signature ______________________

TIME																				COMMENTS
Metaraminol																				
Atropine																				
Bicarbonate																				
Calcium																				
Epinephrine																				
Isoproterenol																				
Levarterenol																				
Lidocaine																				
500 ml. 5% D/W																				
Pupils																				
Pulse																				
Blood pressure																				
Defibrillator DC setting																				

(4) Draw up and label medications as needed. Hand to physician as requested.
(5) Note the medications, amount of medications, and times given to patient, on the cardiac arrest record.
(6) Obtain equipment from emergency cart and hand to physician as needed.
(7) Complete the cardiac arrest sheet and place with patient's record at end of arrest.
(8) At the end of the procedure complete the nursing notes, intravenous therapy sheet, and intake and output record.

b. Second-nurse responsibilities
(1) Assist in cardiopulmonary resuscitation as needed.
(2) Check intubation equipment before handing it to the physician and assist in intubation as needed.
(3) Suction patient.
(4) Take vital signs.
(5) Hang intravenous fluids and regulate drip.
(6) Assist in obtaining blood gases.
(7) Assist in placement of transvenous pacemaker if indicated.

Delivery of drugs by conveyor

When a drug order is transcribed by the unit secretary, she will send the order form (white, yellow, and green copies) to the pharmacy.

The pharmacy will return the white and green copies with the filled prescription. The person removing the medication from the conveyor shall be responsible for signing these copies, which are used as a receipt of medication. The white copy is returned to the pharmacy by return conveyor and the green copy is retained on the floor.

Diabetic control record (Fig. 10)

PURPOSE: To provide a summary of the double-voided and/or fractional urine test results, the corresponding insulin coverage, and the daily weights.

PROCEDURE:

1. To record the results of the urine test, chart in the appropriate column as described.

   Date: Write month, day, and year (example, 7/6/71).

   Time: Specify hour when tested and whether A.M. or P.M. (examples, 7^A, $9{:}30^P$).

   Sugar: Chart results, marking as neg (negative), tr (trace), 1+, 2+, 3+, 4+.

   Acetone: Chart results, labeling as sm (small), mod (moderate), lrg (large), neg (negative).

   Amt. (amount): Record the total amount of the specimen tested (examples, 20 ml., 300 ml.).

2. To record the insulin therapy, chart in the appropriate columns as described.

DIABETIC CONTROL RECORD — Jane Doe 205'

URINE TEST		Doubled Voided and/or Fractional			INSULIN THERAPY						WT.
Date	Time	Sugar	Acetone	Amt. Tested	Time	Type	Dose	Route	Site	Signature	
1-20-73	2^{15} p	2+	neg	30 cc							
1-20-73	4 p	3+	ng	50 cc	4^{45} p	Reg	5 u	SC	RA	P. Green RN	110 lb
1-20-73	9 p	1+	neg	50 cc							
1-21-73	7 A	TR	neg	20 cc							
1-21-73	11 A	1+	neg	25 cc							
1-21-73	4 p	unobtainable									
1-21-73	6 p	1+	neg	20 cc							
1-21-73	9 p	2+	neg	150 cc							
1-22-73	7 A	4+	Sm	20 cc	7^{45} A	Reg	10 u	Sc	LT	P. Green	110

Fig. 10

Time: Specify hour given and whether A.M. or P.M. (examples, 7^A, 12^N).
Type: Write in the kind of insulin given (examples, regular, NPH).
Dose: Number of units given.
Route: Subcutaneous (SC or Subq.); intravenous (IV).
Site: Injection site (see Figs. 13 to 15 for various injections and for acceptable sites).
Signature: First initial, last name, and status (R.N., L.P.N.).

3. To record *daily weights* for the diabetic, chart as indicated.

a. Write in weight, specifying whether lb. or kg., opposite the appropriate time (usually the time when the 7 A.M. double-voided specimen is obtained).
b. Weights done on diabetics should be recorded on this control record daily.

Discharge planning

1. Discharge planning should be started as soon as the physician can predict the possible outcome of medical intervention. Such planning should give attention to these items—as goals:
   a. To restore to optimal health.
   b. To promote continued improvement.
   c. To prevent future complications.
   d. To maintain the level of health achieved.
2. The physician, nurse, and social worker should be in contact and should discuss any need for extended care facilities or family assistance in planning.
3. The complete discharge planning is to be documented in the nursing care plan.
4. Discharge orders should be written 24 hours prior to probable discharge.
5. All discharge orders should include the following:
   a. Medication orders if needed.
   b. Clinic or office visit orders if indicated.
   c. Dietary orders.
   d. Directions concerning extent of activity.
   e. VNA or other referral if needed.
   f. Hospital nursing service follow-up if indicated.
   g. If the patient is to remain in the hospital beyond the discharge hour (11 A.M.) for dressings, laboratory reports, etc., the doctor should make this notation in his discharge orders.
6. The hospital's social service worker will plan for ambulance service when required.
7. When a patient is to be transferred to another hospital or to a nursing home, a brief synopsis, including condition and immediate physician orders, should accompany the patient.
8. If the patient is to receive medications that are presently being dispensed on the unit, the container in use should be sent to the pharmacy and a new prescription be written. All prescriptions may be filled at an outside pharmacy, or the family may take the prescription to the pharmacy in the hospital and purchase the drug on an outpatient basis.
9. Discharge prescriptions are not to be given to the patient by anyone other than the physician, a pharmacist, or an R.N. The purpose of this restriction is to ensure adequate instructions and safety.

Discharge procedure

PURPOSES:

1. To discharge the patient with all possible safety, consideration, and courtesy.

2. To adequately instruct the patient concerning "follow-up care."
3. To complete the chart.

POINTS OF EMPHASIS:

1. The physician will be encouraged to write the order for discharge 24 hours prior to discharge.
2. Planning will be done before the day of discharge.

PROCEDURE:

1. Check the order for discharge. The order must be written by a physician.
2. The unit manager or unit secretary will check with the patient or family concerning transportation and will assist in planning if indicated.
3. The unit manager or unit secretary will complete the discharge slip and will instruct the patient or family member in clearing with the cashier. This may be done in one of two ways:
   a. The family member may take the discharge slip to the cashier and clear for the patient prior to discharge.
   b. The patient may take the discharge slip and clear with the cashier's office as he leaves the hospital.
4. The team leader (R.N.) will complete the discharge instructions. All medication on the hall will be sent back to the pharmacy. A new prescription for any discharge medications will be given to the patient and explained. The nurse or designate will assist the patient in dressing and will notify the unit manager when the patient is ready to leave the hospital.
5. The unit manager or secretary will give the patient an office or clinic appointment slip, if appropriate, and explain.
6. The unit manager will assist the patient in packing all property. He will ascertain if valuables were placed in the safe in the admitting office and see that patient picks them up as he clears the cashier's office.
7. The unit manager or unit secretary will call a transporter to take the patient to the cashier's office and then to his car. The patient will be assisted in getting into his car. If a transporter is not available, this responsibility rests with a member of the nursing staff.
8. The team leader will complete the bedside notes.
9. The unit manager will notify the admitting office that the bed is empty.
10. The unit manager will obtain a discharge diagnosis on the face sheet before the chart is placed in the discharge basket.
11. The unit secretary will remove the patient's name from the dietary slip. She will enter the discharge on the midnight census.
12. The chart will be picked up by the medical records department no later than 9 A.M. of the day after discharge.

Care of patient with external catheter (urosheath)

PURPOSES: To provide a control for urine drainage; to prevent urinary incontinence.

POINT OF EMPHASIS: An external catheter is not meant to be a labor-saving device. It is used when all other means to keep the patient's bed dry—positioning of urinal, offering the patient the urinal every hour until a routine has been established, etc.—have failed. The professional nurse and/or physician should determine the need for the use of an external catheter.

PROCEDURE:

1. Obtain order from physician for external catheter.
2. Order external catheter from central service. Sizes available are medium and large.
3. Apply external catheter according to directions on box.
4. The external catheter will be checked every 4 hours by the team leader, charge nurse, or person assigned to give care (R.N. or L.P.N.)—for adequate drainage of urine.
5. The external catheter will be removed and the physician notified if any of the following conditions are present:
   a. Swelling of penis.
   b. Discoloration of penis.
   c. Any signs of excoriation of penis.
6. The external catheter must be removed for at least ½ hour b.i.d. (for example, 9^{A} and 9^{P}); at these times perineal care is given and the external catheter is washed and dried.
7. Perineal care includes washing the penis and scrotum with warm water and medication as ordered, rinsing well, and drying completely.
8. The perineal care, observation of penis, and care given external catheter are to be charted in the nurses' notes on every shift.
9. Either the treatment section or the special needs section of the Kardex indicates the specific times that the external catheter is to be checked and the times for perineal care.

Incidents

The incident report is to be made in single copy and sent to the nursing service office.

DEFINITION AND PROCEDURE: An incident is any happening that is not consistent with the routine operation of the hospital.

PATIENTS: An incident report shall be filled out on each of the following: fall, injury of any type, use of wrong medication, decubitus ulcer that develops in the hospital, infection, or wrong treatment. The report shall be filled out by a nurse and signed. The physician will also make a report and sign it. All previously ordered activity will be discontinued until the doctor has examined the patient. An x-ray film for possible fracture may be ordered without cost to the patient. The incident report shall be sent to the nursing service office within a 24-hour period.

PERSONNEL: Any employee who is involved shall be sent with the incident report to the emergency room immediately after an incident, whether there is visible injury or not. The employee shall be seen by the emergency room doctor and treated according to his needs. No charge will be made provided the employee goes to the emergency room prior to leaving for home. If the employee suffers an incident to which there are no witnesses and fails to report the incident before leaving the hospital, his subsequent claims for hospital-acquired injuries shall be void. If the employee refuses to go to the emergency room following a reported incident, a note to this effect shall be entered on the incident report. No employee is to be seen by a physician on the nursing unit.

VISITORS AND TRADESMEN: The policy, as it applies to personnel, shall be followed also for visitors or other persons who have a legitimate reason for being in the hospital.

Incident report and safety measures (Fig. 11)

PURPOSES: To record or to prevent occurrence of an incident, which is any happening that is not consistent with the routine operation of the hospital.

PRECAUTIONS AND POINTS OF EMPHASIS:

1. All confused or sedated patients must have side rails up.
2. Know the fire safety regulations (see manual for fire emergency plan).
3. Know the hospital's disaster plan and mass casualty procedure (see manual for disaster plan).
4. Drugs: All medication containers must have clear, unaltered labels.
5. Radioactive substances: Materials that are radioactive must be kept in special labeled containers provided for that purpose.
6. Ether: Open cans of ether or glass containers of ether may not be kept on the nursing unit.
7. Equipment: Malfunctioning equipment constitutes a dangerous hazard and must not be used at any time. Report to the proper department for medical equipment repair.
8. Extension cords: Cords must always be inspected before use.
9. Christmas trees: Refer to policy of hospital pertaining to Christmas decorations.
10. Smoking: Nursing personnel may smoke in the washroom, head nurse station, or cafeteria.
11. Patients may not smoke under the.following circumstances:
    a. When oxygen or other gas is either in use or on standby.
    b. When the patient is alone following sedation.
    c. When patient is irrational or irresponsible and alone.
    d. When in a double room where the other patient is seriously disturbed by the smoke (respiratory distress, allergy, etc.)
    e. When the doctor has forbidden smoking.
12. Open flames: Open flames may be used in the small laboratory on the hall. When sacraments are administered, the lighted candles are not to enter the patient's room.
13. Disposal: Two containers are located in the utility room for disposal of waste material.

a. A large can with a cover is provided for trash and waste that can be burned. Dressings from wounds are wrapped in paper and discarded in the trash can. Do not discard boxes of trash or other material without inspecting for equipment.

b. The second can in the utility room is for glass and metal discards. No cans containing ether or any type of combustible material should be discarded in the trash can; these should be given to the housekeeping personnel to dispose of.

INCIDENT REPORT

"An incident is any happening which is not consistent with the routine operation of the hospital or the routine care of a particular patient. It may be an accident or a situation which might result in an accident."

PERSON INVOLVED

(LAST NAME) (FIRST NAME) (MIDDLE INITIAL)

MR. ☐; MRS. ☐; CHILD ☐; MALE ☐; FEMALE ☐; AGE ______

PATIENT ☐
ROOM NO. | STATE CAUSE FOR HOSPITALIZATION
PATIENT'S CONDITION BEFORE INCIDENT
NORMAL ☐; SENILE ☐; DISORIENTED ☐; SEDATED ☐; OTHER
WERE BED RAILS PRESENT
YES ☐; NO ☐; UP ☐; DOWN ☐; ORDERED ☐
WAS HEIGHT OF BED ADJUSTABLE
YES ☐; NO ☐; UP ☐; DOWN ☐

EMPLOYEE ☐
DEPARTMENT | JOB TITLE

VISITOR ☐
OTHER ☐
HOME ADDRESS | HOME PHONE
OCCUPATION | REASON FOR PRESENCE AT THE HOSPITAL

EXACT LOCATION OF INCIDENT | DATE OF INCIDENT | TIME OF INCIDENT ☐ A.M. ☐ P.M.

PROPERTY INVOLVED ☐; EQUIPMENT INVOLVED ☐; DESCRIBE

DESCRIPTION OF INCIDENT .Y PERSON INVOLVED

DESCRIBE EXACTLY WHAT HAPPENED: WHY IT HAPPENED: WHAT CAUSES WERE. IF AN INJURY, STATE PART OF BODY INJURED. IF PROPERTY OR EQUIPMENT DAMAGED, DESCRIBE DAMAGE.

[illegible] ADDRESS & PHONE NO. OF WITNESS(ES)

WAS PERSON INVOLVED SEEN BY A PHYSICIAN
YES ☐ NO ☐
TIME SEEN ☐ A.M. ☐ P.M.
WHERE

PHYSICIAN'S NAME

STATEMENT OF PHYSICIAN:

DATE OF REPORT | TITLE & SIGNATURE OF PERSON PREPARING REPORT

ADDITIONAL COMMENTS:

Fig. 11

14. Fire doors must remain closed at all times.
15. All spills should be cleaned up immediately.
16. Keep the bed in the lower position unless you are doing care.
17. Furniture should be properly arranged with footstools kept under beds when not in use.
18. Follow procedure principles to avoid errors.
19. Incident reports are made out for any happenings that are not consistent with routine.

PROCEDURE: An incident report is to be made in single copy for the nursing service office.

PATIENTS: An incident report shall be filled out on the following: fall, injury of any type, use of wrong medication, decubitus ulcer that develops in the hospital, or wrong treatment. The report shall be filled out by a nurse and signed. The physician will also make a report and sign it. All previously ordered activity will be discontinued until the doctor has examined the patient. An x-ray film for possible fracture may be ordered without cost to the patient. The incident report shall be sent to the nursing service office within a 24-hour period.

PERSONNEL: Every employee suffering an accident shall be sent with an incident report to the emergency room immediately after an incident, whether there is visible injury or not. The employee shall be seen by the emergency room doctor and treated according to his needs. No charge will be made provided the employee goes to the emergency room prior to leaving for home. If the employee suffers an incident to which there are no witnesses and fails to report the incident before leaving the hospital, his subsequent claims for hospital-acquired injuries shall be void. If the employee refuses to go to the emergency room following a reported incident, a note to this effect shall be entered on the incident report. No employee is to be seen by a physician on the nursing unit.

VISITORS AND TRADESMEN: The policy, as it applies to personnel, shall be followed also for visitors or other persons who have a legitimate reason for being in the hospital.

Intake and output record (Fig. 12)

PURPOSE: To maintain an accurate and current record of the fluid intake and output balance.

PROCEDURE:

Date: At 7 A.M. each day the 11-7:30 shift begins a new sheet. The date for the 24 hours is written. For instance, at 7 A.M. on Thursday, 2/7/74, the date 2/7/74 is recorded.

A. Intake
   1. Parenteral
      Solution section
      a. When starting parenteral fluids (IV bottle, blood, albumin, Cortland,

hyperalimentation, and piggyback), always write the bottle number and the amount and type of solution.

b. At the end of each shift write, at the beginning of the next shift's section, the bottle number and the amount and type of solution remaining to infuse.

Infused section

a. When a bottle is completed or discontinued, write the correct amount that has infused.

INTAKE AND OUTPUT RECORD

Date: 1-21-73

Mrs. J. Doe 205'

shift	INTAKE				OUTPUT			
	Parenteral		Oral		Urine		Other	
	Solution	Infused	Type	Amount	Source	Amount	Source	Amount
7 a.m. - 3 p.m.	#3 300 cc 5% DIW left #4 500 cc L.R.	300 400	Tube feeding water water water Tube feeding water	200 cc 100 cc 50 cc 50 cc 200 cc 100 cc			Hemovac	200
	8 HOUR TOTALS	700		700	Foley Catheter	1150		200
	BLOOD - 8 HOUR TOTAL							
3 p.m. - 11 p.m.	# 100 cc L.R #1 1000 D5%/L.R #2 1000 cc NS	100 1000 50	water Tea Tube F Water Tea Jello water water water	50 150 200 100 160 100 100 100 100	F. Cath Vd.	900 300	Hemovac Diarrhea stools Hemovac Stool	100 ✓✓✓✓ 150 4 X
	8 HOUR TOTAL	1150		1060		1200	Hemovac	250
	BLOOD - 8 HOUR TOTAL							
11 p.m. - 7 a.m.	#2 950 NS #3 1000 5DIW s̄ 40 mEq KCl.	950 150	water water Tea ice Cream Broth Jello water water	100 100 160 120 100 120 150 100	vd. vd vd	650 700 575	Hemovac Stool Hemovac	100 ✓✓ 50
	8 HOUR TOTAL	1100		950		1925	stool	2X 150
	BLOOD - 8 HOUR TOTAL							
	24 HOUR BLOOD						stool	6 X
	24 HOUR TOTAL	2950		2710		4275	Hemovac	600

Fig. 12

b. At the end of each shift, write the amount infused of the current bottle.
c. The remainder of the parenteral fluid at the end of the shift is written in the next shift's column.

2. Oral section
Type of fluid: Examples, orange juice, milk, tube feeding (T.F.), gastrostomy T.F., tea, ice cream, ice chips, etc.
Amount of fluid: Check the measurement list for guidelines.

B. Output
1. Urine section
Source: Indicate (examples, voided, catheter, ureterostomy, cystostomy, incontinent).
Amount: As measured.
2. Other section
Source: Indicate (examples, nasal-gastric tube, Levin tube, Cantor tube, Salen sump tube, ileo bladder, colostomy, ileostomy, diarrhea stools).
Amount: As measured.

Totals: Done at the end of each shift, and the 24-hour total is done at 7 A.M. Blood will be totaled at the end of each shift, and the 24-hour total will be done at 7 A.M.

Charting: The 11-7:30 shift is responsible for (1) adding the 24-hour totals, (2) recording these totals on the temperature record, and (3) beginning a new intake and output record at 7 A.M.

Injection sites (Figs. 13 to 15)

The charting of injections is of paramount importance. The frequency with which we find ourselves involved with litigation concerning the giving and charting of intramuscular and subcutaneous injections makes it imperative that we not only give injections in the proper site but that we differentiate sites in our charting. Figs. 13 to 15 will assist you.

ABBREVIATIONS FOR CHARTING

Intramuscular sites (gluteus medius)

Key:
R—Right
L—Left
U—Upper
O—Outer
G—Gluteus muscle

RUOG—Right upper outer gluteus
LUOG—Left upper outer gluteus

Ventrogluteal area

R—Right
L—Left
VG—Ventrogluteal

RVG—Right ventrogluteal
LVG—Left ventrogluteal

Mid-deltoid area

R—Right
L—Left
MD—Mid-deltoid

RMD—Right mid-deltoid
LMD—Left mid-deltoid

Text continued on p. 117.

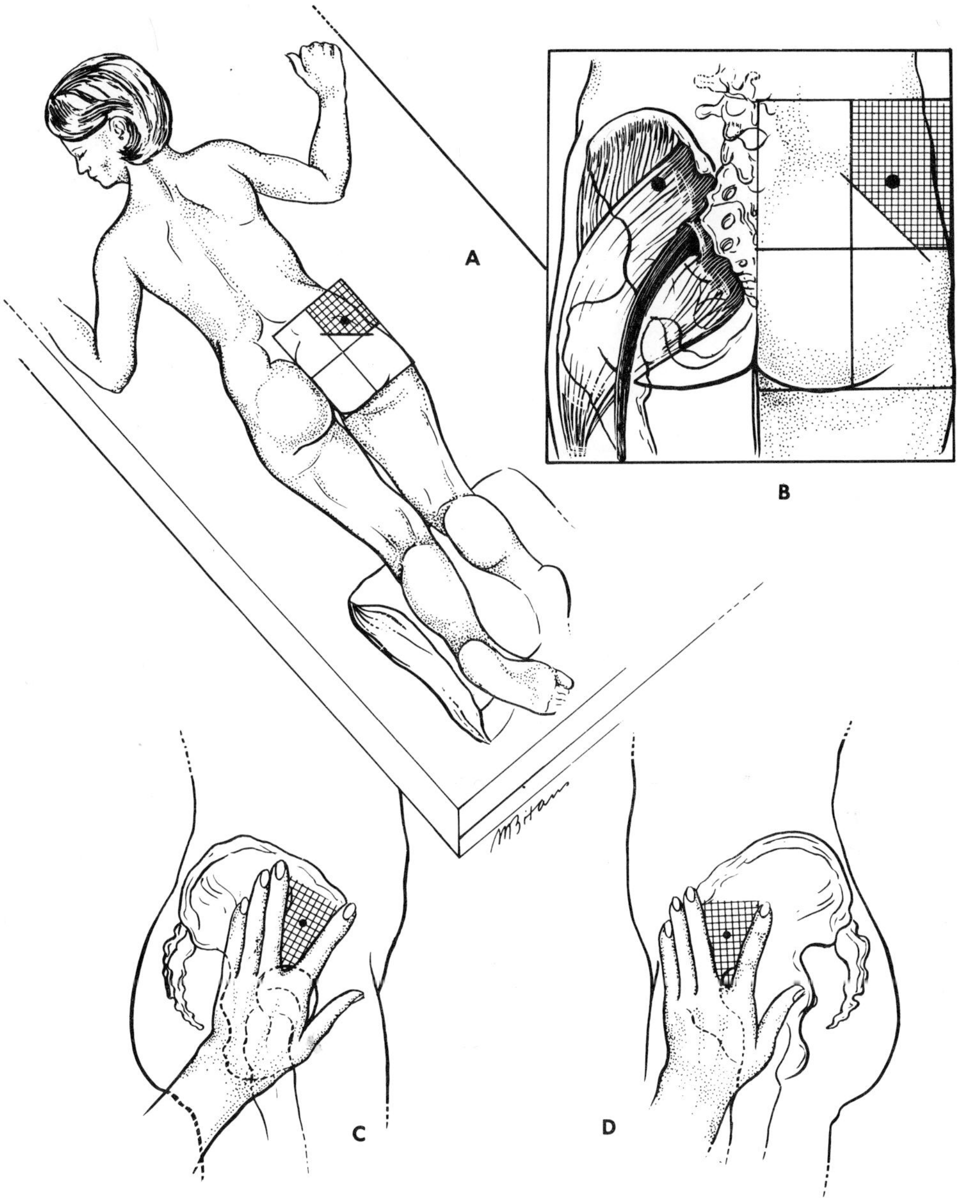

Continued.

Fig. 13. Sites for intramuscular injection. **A,** Position of patient when posterior gluteal area is used. **B,** Diagram showing the anatomy of posterior gluteal area and the method of finding injection site. Large dot indicates site of injection. **C,** Location of site for injection into right ventrogluteal area. **D,** Location of site for injection into left gluteal area. **E** and **F,** Location of boundaries for injection into vastus lateralis. **G** and **H,** Location of site for injection into deltoid. (From Dison, Norma: An atlas of nursing techniques, ed. 2, St. Louis, 1971, The C. V. Mosby Co.)

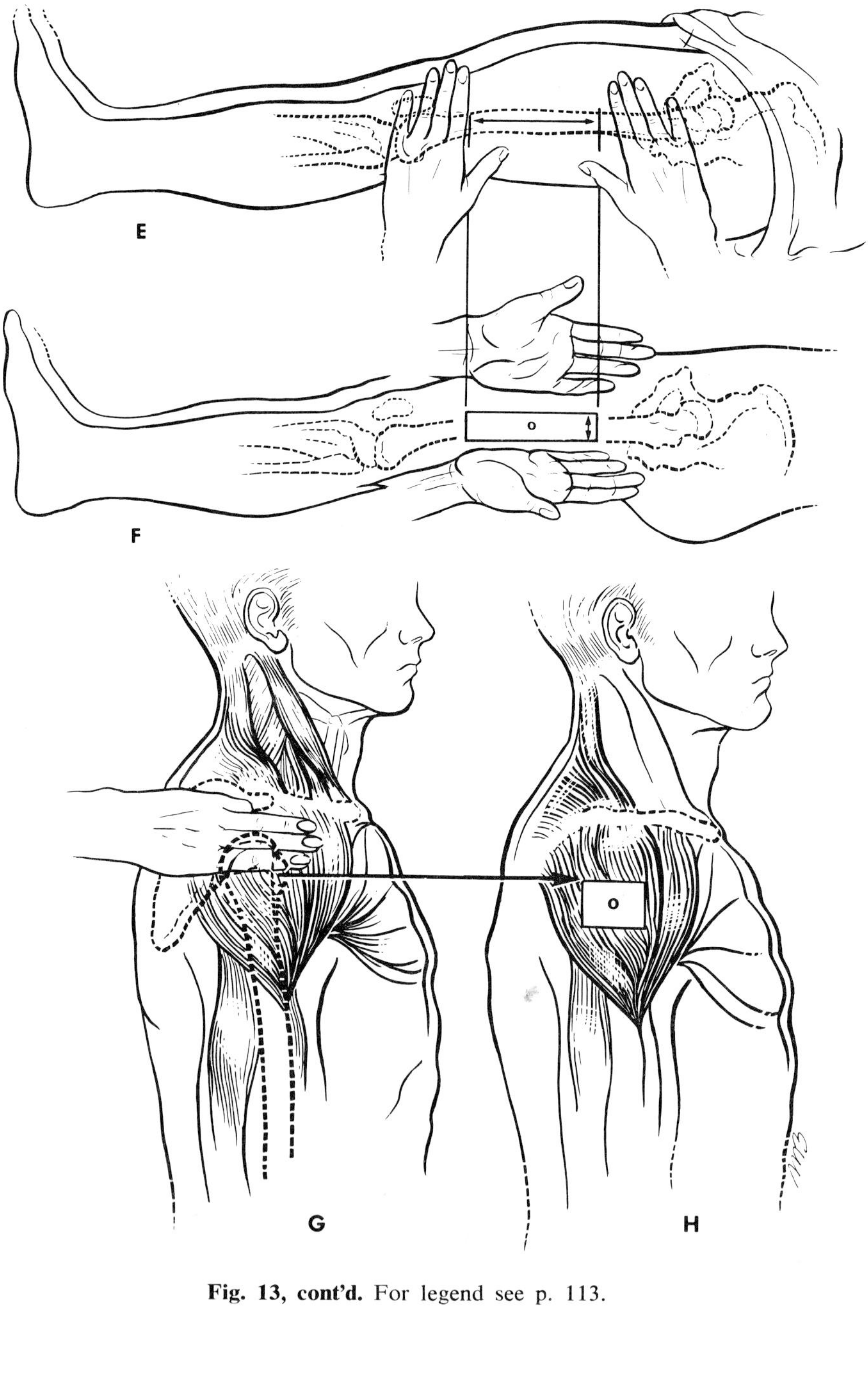

Fig. 13, cont'd. For legend see p. 113.

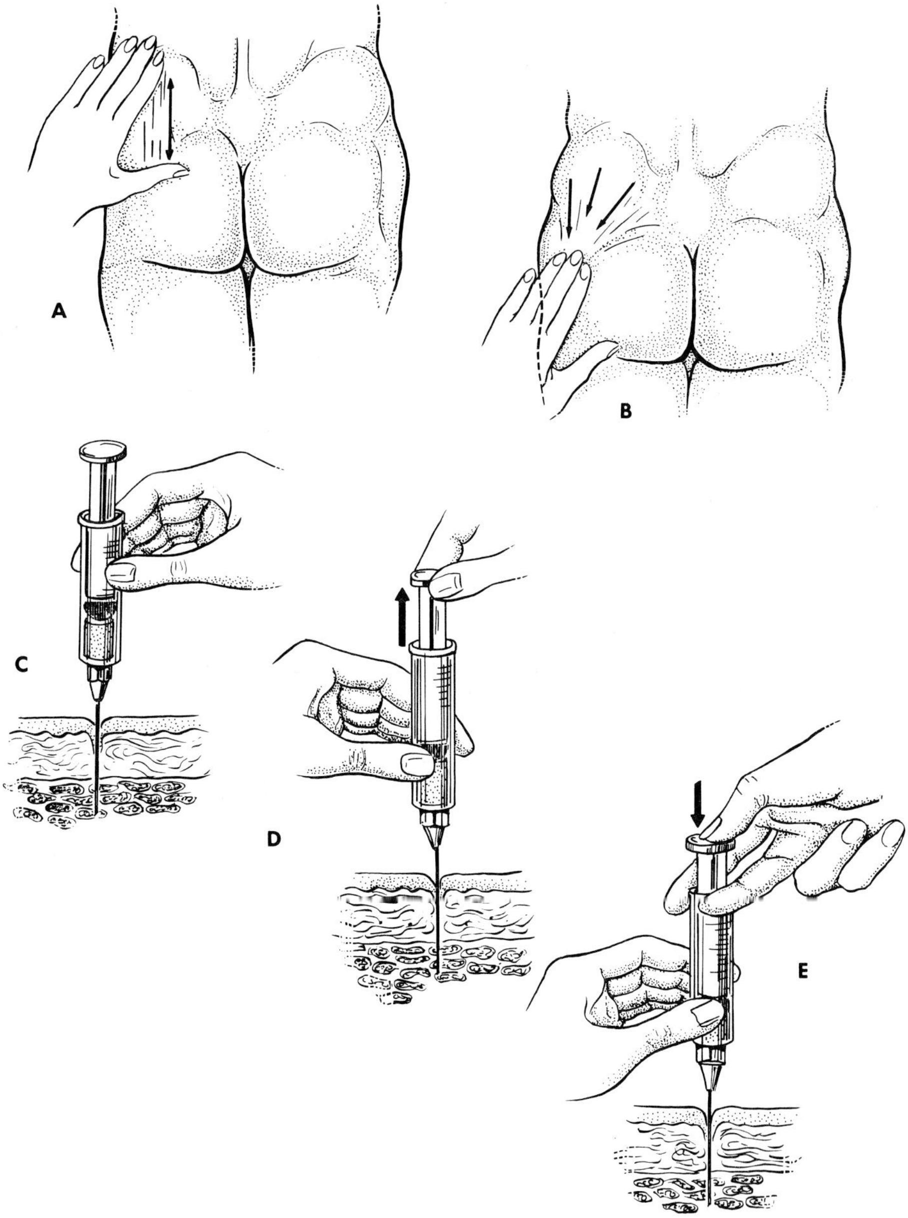

Fig. 14. Technique of intramuscular injection. **A,** One method of stretching tissues. **B,** An alternate method of stretching tissues. **C,** Needle is inserted at right angle to tissues. **D,** Plunger is withdrawn slightly to make certain that needle is not located within a blood vessel. **E,** Solution is injected. (From Dison, Norma: An atlas of nursing techniques, ed. 2, St. Louis, 1971, The C. V. Mosby Co.)

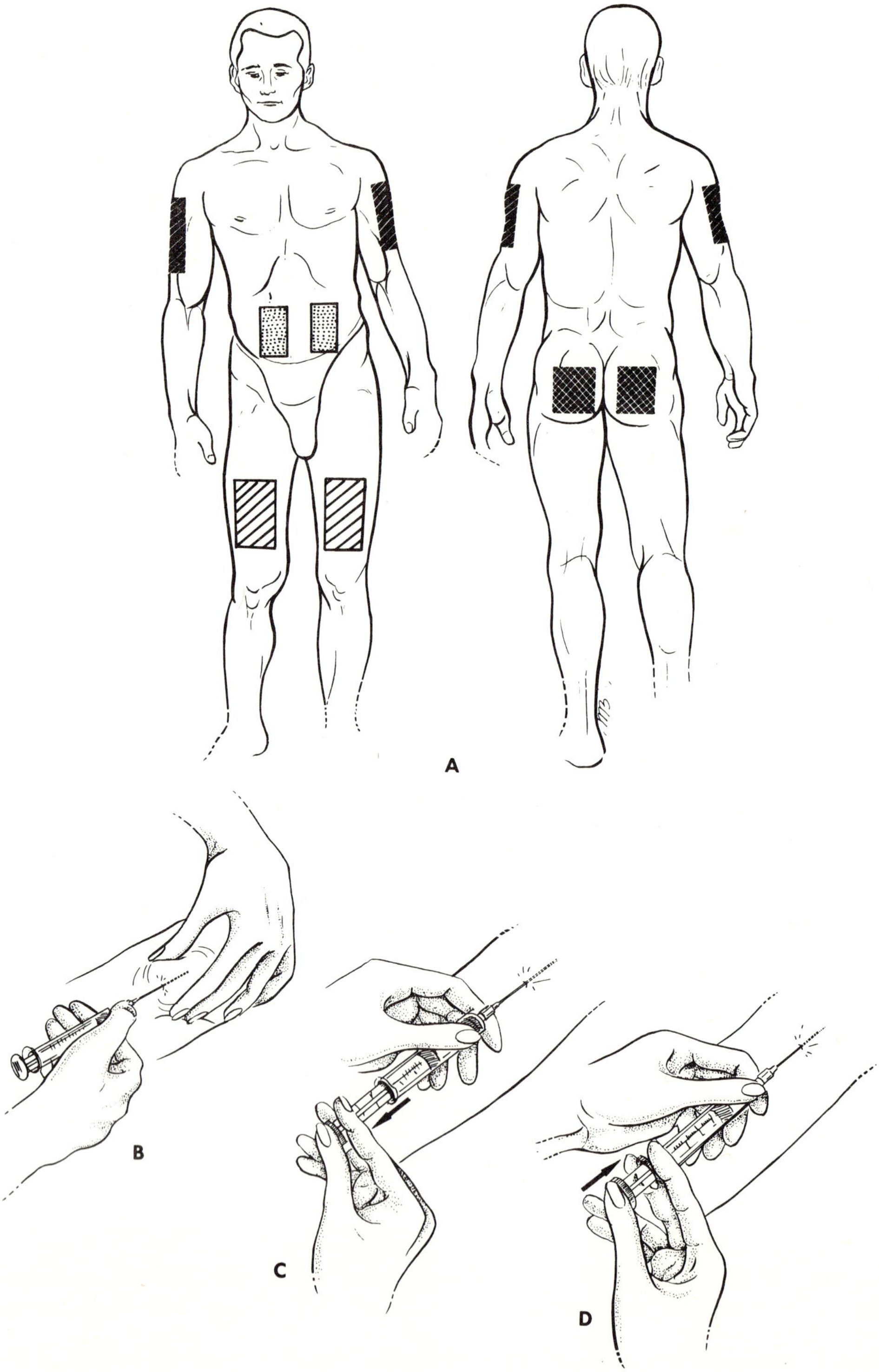

Fig. 15. For legend see opposite page.

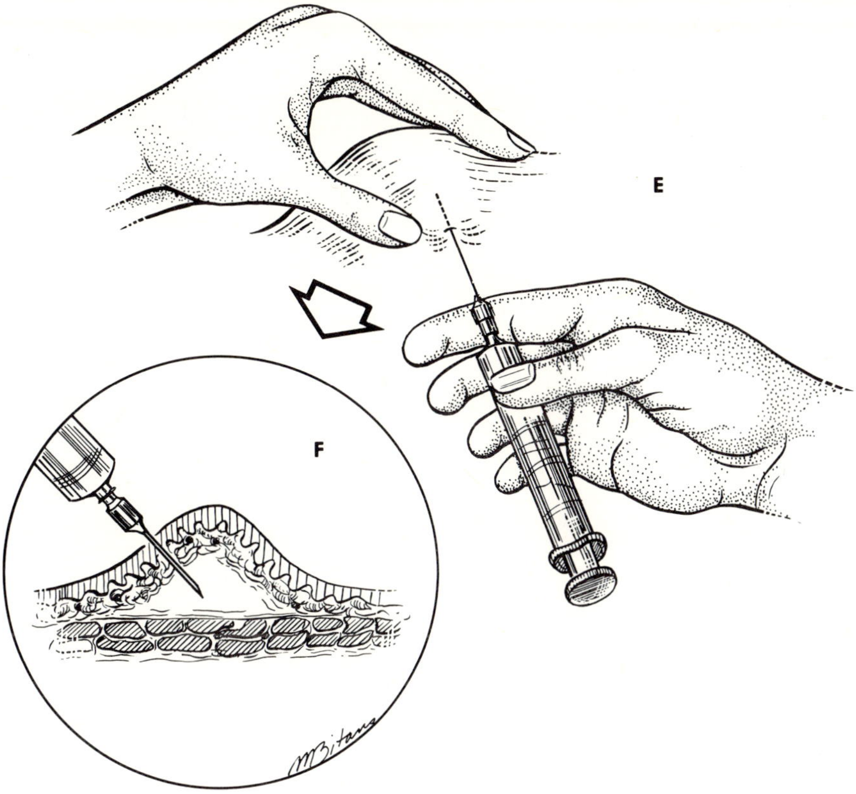

Fig. 15. Subcutaneous injection. **A,** Possible sites for injection. **B,** Method of tensing tissue during insertion of needle. **C,** After insertion of needle, plunger is withdrawn slightly, to determine that needle is not located within a blood vessel. **D,** Drug is injected by pushing plunger forward. **E,** The method of tensing tissue that is used for injection of irritating drugs. **F,** Cross section showing relationship of needle to tissues. (From Dison, Norma: An atlas of nursing techniques, ed. 2, St. Louis, 1971, The C. V. Mosby Co.)

Vastus lateralis

R—Right
L—Left
VL—Vastus lateralis
RVL—Right vastus lateralis
LVL—Left vastus lateralis

Intravenous fluid card (Fig. 16)

PURPOSE: To provide a consistent method of control in meeting the physician's orders for IV fluids, including blood and albumin.

PROCEDURE:

Initiation: The secretary or unit manager transcribes the physician's order as written and makes certain entries on the IV card.

Date: Include day, month, year.

Name: Print patient's full name (example, John Doe).

Room: Include room and bed number.

IV labels: Each daily IV series is to be numbered (example, 1-2-3) or lettered (a-b-c).

I V F L U I D S

DATE: ____________________

NAME: ____________________

ROOM: ____________________

NO.	AMT. - TYPE - ADDITIVES	TIME SPAN	STARTED		AMT. LEFT		
			DATE	TIME	3^P	11^P	7^A

RATE:

Fig. 16

Amount, type, and additives: Complete as written in the physician's order (example, 1000 ml. 5% D/W with 40 mEq. KCL).

Time span: Length of time each bottle is to be infusing (example, 8 hours, 6 hours; KVO—keep vein open).

Rate: Number of milliliters per hour or drops per minute if specified by the physician.

Any special orders may be written in the empty space at the bottom of the card.

Updating: The team leader has the responsibility for completing the following sections:

1. Started: Date and time (example, 1/4, 8^{A}).
2. Amount left: Number of cc. remaining in the IV bottle at the end of each shift is written in the respective column at the change-of-shift report.
3. When one bottle of IV fluids is completed, the team leader draws a line through that order.
4. Calculate and write in the rate if not written by the physician.
5. The IV card is *always* kept in the upper flap of the Kardex.

Infection control standards

PURPOSE: To provide a system that will control and prevent the spread of infection.

IMPLEMENTATION: The request for isolation is initiated by a doctor's order. The order must include

1. Request for isolation with specified type.
2. Reason (diagnosis).

CONTROL: The clinical nurse is responsible for enforcing the standards. Any infraction that cannot be resolved should be brought to the attention of the nursing service representative to the Infection Control Committee.

RESPONSE TO THE ORDER: On receipt of the order for isolation, the *clinical nurse* is responsible for establishing the appropriate technique. A supply of the five different disposable cards (one for each category of isolation and precaution) will be kept at the nurses' station on each floor. After the appropriate technique has been chosen, the *unit manager* will do the following:

1. Place the patient in the appropriate room.
2. Place the precaution card, with the technique to be followed, on the wall above the isolation stand outside the patient's room.
3. Place an isolation sticker on the front of the chart.
4. Place the precaution card with the appropriate disease entity on the inside cover of the chart.
5. Indicate in red on the patient's Kardex the appropriate isolation to be followed.
6. Gather and position the appropriate equipment for the patient's room.
7. Call central service for the specific *isolation pack.*
8. If protective isolation is ordered, check with the physician to determine if sterile linen, gowns, or gloves are needed.

NOTIFICATION: The patient, his family, and specific departments within the hospital will be notified of the patient's need for isolation precaution.

Physician's responsibilities

1. Informing the patient of the need to place him on isolation.
2. Explaining to family members the need for such procedure.
3. Writing the order requesting the appropriate technique.

Clinical nurse's responsibilities

1. Reviewing with the patient the need for instituting such precautions.
2. Informing and teaching the patient specific ways in which he can enhance the efficacy of the procedure.
3. Instructing the family members concerning the appropriate protocol to be followed.
4. Informing nursing personnel that the patient is on isolation.
5. Instructing nursing personnel in the rationale and techniques of isolation precautions.
6. Checking the patient's room to see that the equipment is appropriately placed and used.
7. Informing nursing personnel that they are responsible for delivery of *all* isolation trays as well as for picking up the trays of *all* isolation patients. The regular trays will be placed on a cart in the floor kitchen. The disposable trays will be placed in the trash barrels inside the rooms.

Unit manager's responsibilities

1. Notifying the admitting office if a room change is indicated.

2. Notifying dietary of the need for an isolation disposable tray by indicating on the diet list the type of isolation precaution required.
3. Notifying the visitor's desk of patients who are on isolation as well as notifying them when the patient is taken off isolation.
4. Overseeing that all requisitions are marked "Isolation" so that the ancillary departments can take appropriate precautions.
5. Notifying the housekeeping department that the patient has been placed on isolation and what type.
6. Notifying employee health service by compiling a list of all persons exposed to hepatitis, tuberculosis, etc.

GROUPS:

I. Enteric precautions (Fig. 17)

Enteric Precautions

Visitors—Report to Nurses' Station Before Entering Room

1. **Private Room**—*necessary for children only.*
2. **Gowns**—must be worn by all persons having direct contact with patient.
3. **Masks**—not necessary.
4. **Hands**—must be washed on entering and leaving room.
5. **Gloves**—must be worn by all persons having direct contact with patient or with articles contaminated with fecal material.
6. **Articles**—special precautions necessary for articles contaminated with urine and feces. Articles must be disinfected or discarded.

Diseases Requiring Enteric Precautions*

1. **Cholera**
2. **Enteropathogenic *E. coli* gastroenteritis**
3. **Hepatitis, viral (infectious or serum)**
4. **Salmonellosis (including typhoid fever)**
5. **Shigellosis**

***See *Isolation Techniques for Use in Hospitals* for details and recommended duration of isolation.**

PHS Publication No. 2054-D
For sale by the Superintendent of Documents, U.S. Government Printing Office, Washington, D.C. 20402
Price: 10¢ each or $6.75 per 100

Fig. 17

Purpose: To prevent spread of disease that can be transmitted through direct or indirect contact with infected feces and, in some instances, heavily contaminated articles. Transmission of infection depends on ingestion of the pathogen.

Diseases

1. Cholera
2. Enteropathogenic *E. coli* gastroenteritis
3. Hepatitis, viral (infectious or serum)
4. Salmonellosis (including typhoid fever)
5. Shigellosis

Technique

1. Private room	Door open.
2. Gowns	Must be worn by all persons having direct contact with patient.
3. Masks	*Not* necessary.
4. Hands	*Must* be washed on entering and on leaving room.
5. Gloves	Must be worn by all persons having direct contact with patient or with articles contaminated with fecal material.
6. Articles	Must be double bagged in red plastic bags before removing from room and sending to central service.
7. Linen	Should be placed in trash barrel lined with red linen bag. Must be double bagged in a red linen bag before removing from room and sending to laundry.
8. Trash	Must be double bagged in red plastic bags before removing from room and placing in utility room.
9. Food	An isolation tray must be ordered.
10. Laboratory specimens	Should be double bagged in plastic bags.
11. Transporting the patient	No special precautions are needed unless the patient is incontinent; he should not be moved from the isolation room.
12. Visitors	Should be instructed on the precautions.

Equipment

INSIDE ROOM	OUTSIDE ROOM
Plastic barrel lined with red plastic	Isolation stand
Plastic barrel lined with red linen	Disposable gowns
Hand-washing care	Disposable gloves
Sphygmomanometer	Transparent bags
Stethoscope	Red linen bags
Thermometer	Red plastic bags
Red box for disposable needles	
Isolation food tray must be ordered	

II. Wound and skin precautions (Fig. 18)

Wound & Skin Precautions

Visitors—Report to Nurses' Station Before Entering Room

1. **Private Room**—desirable.
2. **Gowns**—must be worn by all persons having direct contact with patient.
3. **Masks**—not necessary except during dressing changes.
4. **Hands**—must be washed on entering and leaving room.
5. **Gloves**—must be worn by all persons having direct contact with infected area.
6. **Articles**—special precautions necessary for instruments, dressings, and linen.

NOTE: *See* manual for Special Dressing Techniques to be used when changing dressings.

Diseases Requiring Wound & Skin Precautions*

1. **Burns, extensive, not infected with *Staphylococcus aureus* or Group A streptococcus**
2. **Gas gangrene**
3. **Impetigo**
4. **Staphylococcal skin and wound infections**
5. **Streptococcal skin infection**
6. **Wound infection, extensive**

***See *Isolation Techniques for Use in Hospitals* for details and recommended duration of isolation.**

PHS Publication No. 2054-E
For sale by the Superintendent of Documents, U.S. Government Printing Office, Washington, D.C. 20402
Price: 10¢ each or $6.75 per 100

Fig. 18

Purpose: To prevent cross-infection of personnel and patients from infection transmissible by direct contact with wounds and heavily contaminated articles.

Diseases

1. Burns, extensive, *not* infected with staphylococci or streptococci
2. Gas gangrene
3. Impetigo
4. Staphylococcal skin and wound infection
5. Streptococcal skin infection
6. Wound infection, extensive

Technique

1. Private room Door open.

2. Gowns	Must be worn by all persons having direct contact with patients.
3. Masks	*Not* necessary *except* during dressing changes.
4. Hands	Must be washed on entering and on leaving room.
5. Gloves	Must be worn by all persons having direct contact with *infected* area.
6. Articles	If the item has come in direct contact with the *infected* area, it should be double bagged in red plastic bags before sending to central service.
7. Linen	Should be placed in trash barrel lined with red linen bag. Must be double bagged in a red linen bag before removing from room and sending to laundry.
8. Trash	Must be double bagged in red plastic bags before removing from room and placing in utility room.
9. Food	No special precautions.
10. Laboratory specimens	No special precautions.
11. Transporting the patient	The infected area should be covered with a sterile barrier towel.
12. Visitors	Should be instructed on the precautions.

Equipment

INSIDE ROOM	OUTSIDE ROOM
Plastic barrel lined with red plastic	Isolation stand
Plastic barrel lined with red linen	Disposable gowns
Hand-washing cart	Disposable gloves
Sphygmomanometer	Disposable masks
Stethoscope	Red linen bags
Thermometer	Red plastic bags
Red box for disposable needles	Transparent bags

III. Respiratory isolation (Fig. 19)

Purpose: To prevent transmission of organisms by means of droplets and droplet nuclei that are coughed, sneezed, or breathed into the environment. Also, some of the organisms responsible for illnesses listed in this category can be spread by freshly contaminated articles.

Diseases

1. Chickenpox
2. Herpes zoster
3. Measles (rubeola)
4. Meningococcal meningitis
5. Meningococcemia
6. Mumps
7. Pertussis (whooping cough)
8. Rubella (German measles)

Respiratory Isolation

Visitors—Report to Nurses' Station Before Entering Room

1. **Private Room**—*necessary*; door must be kept closed.
2. **Gowns**—not necessary.
3. **Masks**—must be worn by all persons entering room if susceptible to disease.
4. **Hands**—must be washed on entering and leaving room.
5. **Gloves**—not necessary.
6. **Articles**—those contaminated with secretions must be disinfected.
7. **Caution**—all persons susceptible to the specific disease should be excluded from patient area; if contact is necessary, susceptibles must wear masks.

Diseases Requiring Respiratory Isolation*

1. **Chickenpox**
2. **Herpes zoster**
3. **Measles (rubeola)**
4. **Meningococcal meningitis**
5. **Meningococcemia**
6. **Mumps**
7. **Pertussis (whooping cough)**
8. **Rubella (German measles)**
9. **Tuberculosis, pulmonary—sputum-positive (or suspect)**
10. **Venezuelan equine encephalomyelitis**

***See *Isolation Techniques for Use in Hospitals* for details and recommended duration of isolation.**

PHS Publication No. 2054-B
For sale by the Superintendent of Documents, U.S. Government Printing Office, Washington, D.C. 20402
Price: 10¢ each or $6.75 per 100

Fig. 19

9. Tuberculosis, pulmonary sputum positive (or suspect)
10. Venezuelan equine encephalomyelitis

Technique

1. Private room	Equipped with ultraviolet lights, door open.
2. Gowns	Not necessary.
3. Masks	*Not* needed *unless* patient is unable to cover mouth when coughing or sneezing.
4. Hands	Must be washed on entering and on leaving room.
5. Gloves	Not necessary.
6. Articles	Those contaminated with secretions should be double bagged in red plastic bags and sent to central service.

7. Linen	No special precautions.
8. Trash	Must be double bagged in red plastic bags before removing from room and placing in utility room.
9. Food	No special precautions.
10. Laboratory specimens	No special precautions.
11. Transporting the patient	The patient should wear a disposable mask when out of the room.
12. Visitors	The patient should wear a mask when visitors are present.

Equipment

INSIDE ROOM	OUTSIDE ROOM
Wastebasket lined with red plastic	Isolation stand
Hand-washing cart	Disposable masks
Sphygmomanometer	Six brown paper bags
Stethoscope	Red plastic bags
Thermometer	
Brown paper bag attached to bed	

IV. Strict isolation (Fig. 20)

Purpose: To prevent the transmission of all highly communicable diseases that are spread by both contact and airborne routes of transmission.

Diseases

1. Anthrax, inhalation
2. Burns, extensive, infected with *Staphylococcus aureus* or with Group A streptococci
3. Diphtheria
4. Eczema vaccinatum
5. Melioidosis, pulmonary, or extrapulmonary with draining sinus(es)
6. Herpes simplex
7. Plague
8. Rabies
9. Rubella (German measles) and congenital rubella syndrome
10. Smallpox
11. Staphylococcal enterocolitis
12. Staphylococcal pneumonia
13. Streptococcal pneumonia
14. Vaccinia, generalized and progressive

Technique

1. Private room	Door must be kept closed.
2. Gowns	Must be worn by all persons entering patient's room.
3. Masks	Must be worn by all persons entering patient's room.
4. Hands	Must be washed on entering and on leaving room.
5. Gloves	Must be worn by all persons entering patient's room.

Strict Isolation

Visitors—Report to Nurses' Station Before Entering Room

1. **Private Room**—*necessary*; door must be kept closed.
2. **Gowns**—must be worn by all persons entering room.
3. **Masks**—must be worn by all persons entering room.
4. **Hands**—must be washed on entering and leaving room.
5. **Gloves**—must be worn by all persons entering room.
6. **Articles**—must be discarded, or wrapped before being sent to Central Supply for disinfection or sterilization.

Diseases Requiring Strict Isolation*

1. **Anthrax, inhalation**
2. **Burns, extensive, infected with *Staphylococcus aureus* or Group A streptococcus**
3. **Diphtheria**
4. **Eczema vaccinatum**
5. **Melioidosis, pulmonary, or extra-pulmonary with draining sinus(es)**
6. **Neonatal vesicular disease (Herpes simplex)**
7. **Plague**
8. **Rabies**
9. **Rubella (German measles) and Congenital rubella syndrome**
10. **Smallpox**
11. **Staphylococcal enterocolitis**
12. **Staphylococcal pneumonia**
13. **Streptococcal pneumonia**
14. **Vaccinia, generalized and progressive**

***See *Isolation Techniques for Use in Hospitals* for details and recommended duration of isolation.**

PHS Publication No. 2054-A
For sale by the Superintendent of Documents, U.S. Government Printing Office, Washington, D.C. 20402
Price: 10¢ each or $6.75 per 100

Fig. 20

6. Articles	Must be discarded or double bagged in red plastic bag before being sent to central service.
7. Linen	Should be placed in trash barrel lined with red linen bag. Must be double bagged in red linen bag before removing from room and sending to laundry.
8. Trash	Must be double bagged in red plastic bags before removing from room and placing in utility room.
9. Food	An isolation tray must be ordered.
10. Laboratory specimens	Should be double bagged in plastic bags.
11. Transporting the patient	The patient should wear an isolation gown as well as mask and gloves. A clean cotton blanket should be

placed over the stretcher or wheelchair and then wrapped around the patient.

12. Visitors	Should be limited to two at a time. Before entering room, visitors should be instructed in the use of gowns, masks, and gloves.

Equipment

INSIDE ROOM	OUTSIDE ROOM
Plastic barrel lined with red plastic	Isolation stand
Plastic barrel lined with red linen	Disposable gowns
Wastebasket lined with red plastic	Disposable gloves
Hand-washing cart	Disposable masks
Sphygmomanometer	Plastic bags
Stethoscope	Red linen bags
Thermometer	Red plastic bags
Red box for disposable needles	Brown paper bags
Isolation food tray as ordered	
Brown paper bag on bed	

V. Protective isolation (Fig. 21)

Purpose: To prevent contact between potentially pathogenic microorganisms (including commensal microorganisms) and uninfected persons who have seriously impaired resistance.

Diseases and/or patients

1. Agranulocytosis
2. Severe and extensive, noninfected vesicular, bullous, or eczematous dermatitis
3. Certain patients receiving immunosuppressive therapy
4. Certain patients with lymphomas and leukemia
5. Burned patients (not infected)

Technique

1. Private room	*Necessary.* Door must be kept closed.
2. Gowns	Must be worn by all persons entering room.
3. Masks	Must be worn by all persons entering room.
4. Hands	Must be washed on entering and on leaving room.
5. Gloves	Must be worn by all persons having direct contact with patient.
6. Articles	No special precautions.
7. Linen	Check with physician to see if sterile linens are necessary.
8. Trash	No special precautions.
9. Food	Regular tray may be used.
10. Laboratory specimens	No special precautions.
11. Transporting the patient	Should be curtailed to avoid exposure to any source of infection.

Protective Isolation

Visitors—Report to Nurses' Station Before Entering Room

1. **Private Room**—*necessary*; door must be kept closed.
2. **Gowns**—must be worn by all persons entering room.
3. **Masks**—must be worn by all persons entering room.
4. **Hands**—must be washed on entering and leaving room.
5. **Gloves**—must be worn by all persons having direct contact with patient.
6. **Articles**—*see* manual text.

Conditions Requiring Protective Isolation*

1. **Agranulocytosis**
2. **Severe and extensive, noninfected vesicular, bullous, or eczematous dermatitis**
3. **Certain patients receiving immunosuppressive therapy**
4. **Certain patients with lymphomas and leukemia**

***See *Isolation Techniques for Use in Hospitals* for details and recommended duration of isolation.**

PHS Publication No. 2054-C
For sale by the Superintendent of Documents, U.S. Government Printing Office, Washington, D.C. 20402
Price: 10¢ each or $6.75 per 100

Fig. 21

12. Visitors — Visitors should be instructed in the use of gowns, masks, and gloves.

Equipment

INSIDE ROOM	OUTSIDE ROOM
Thermometer	Isolation stand
Stethoscope	Hand-washing cart
Sphygmomanometer	Gowns (optional, sterile)
	Masks
	Gloves, sterile
	Linen (optional, sterile)
	Regular tray
	Plastic barrel for trash

Isolation equipment from central service

DEFINITION: Essential items are issued by central service for establishing and maintaining isolation precautions.

PROCEDURE:

1. Physician will write order for isolation.
2. Clinical nurse or designate will indicate which group.
3. Unit manager or designate will order isolation equipment and specific pack from central service by indicating the group.
4. Central service will respond by always sending
   a. Hand-washing cart
   b. Isolation stand
   c. Specific isolation equipment
5. Nursing personnel are responsible for cleaning all equipment before sending it back to central service.
6. Unit manager will be responsible for sending all equipment back to central service when the isolation precautions are terminated.

EQUIPMENT: The type of equipment will vary according to the group specified.

Group I: Enteric precautions

Two plastic cans
Pack
- Stethoscope
- Thermometer
- Red box for disposable needles
- Twenty disposable gowns
- One box of disposable gloves
- Two dozen transparent bags

Group II: Wound and skin precautions

Two plastic cans
Pack
- Stethoscope
- Thermometer
- Red box for disposable needles
- Twenty disposable gowns
- One box of disposable gloves
- One box of disposable masks
- Two dozen transparent bags

Group III: Respiratory isolation

Pack
- Stethoscope
- Thermometer
- One box of disposable masks

Group IV: Strict isolation

Two plastic cans
Pack

Stethoscope
Thermometer
Red box for disposable needles
Twenty disposable gowns
One box of disposable gloves
One box of disposable masks
Two dozen transparent bags

Group V: Protective isolation

One plastic can
Pack
Stethoscope
Thermometer
One box of disposable masks
Twenty disposable gowns
One box of sterile gloves
Optional (check with unit manager)
Sterile gowns } Floor should provide linen that needs to be sterilized.
Sterile linen }

NOTE: Red plastic bags will be floor stock on each unit. Red linen bags can be ordered from the linen department. Unit manager should assess needs for 24-hour supply of isolation equipment and order accordingly from central service daily by 2 P.M.

Hand-washing cart

PURPOSE: To provide hand-washing facilities where a permanent facility is not available.

USES:

The hand-washing cart can be ordered for

1. Patients in isolation.
2. Patients who do not have sink facilities.
3. Provision of additional sink facilities.

EQUIPMENT:

Portable cart
Two dispensers with foot controls
Towel rack with paper towels
Aluminum basin
Liquid soap
Water

RESPONSIBILITIES:

Central service

1. Storage of carts
2. Assembling of carts
3. Delivery to unit

4. Terminal cleaning

Patient services

1. Ordering of cart
2. Charging of cart
3. Proper placement of cart
4. Removal and return of cart, when need no longer exists.

Housekeeping

1. Adding towels while cart is in use.
2. Adding new soap and water while cart is in use.
3. Cleaning cart while in use.
4. Wiping cart and emptying towel rack and bottles before it is sent to central service.

Nursing service

1. Emptying basin at the end of every shift or as necessary.
2. Checking to see that soap and water dispensers and towel rack are filled and, if not, filling them.

TERMINAL ISOLATION CLEANING PROCEDURES

EQUIPMENT:

Germicidal solution
Toilet bowl swab
Small bucket
Large bucket
Clean rags
Mop
Cleanser
Toilet tissue, paper towels, liquid soap
Ultraviolet lights (2)
Cubicle curtains
Linen

RESPONSIBILITY:

Housekeeping personnel are responsible for cleaning and making the patient area acceptable for a new patient.

Nursing unit is responsible for all the medical equipment in the patient's room, including removing and replacing the sphygmomanometer covering.

Patient service department will see that the equipment is returned to the appropriate department and will order a new cover for sphygmomanometer.

PROCEDURE:

1. Before entering room to be cleaned, put on isolation gown, mask, and gloves.
2. Raise head and foot of bed.
3. Open all drawers, doors to closets and to connecting bath, remove toilet tissue, paper hand towels.
4. Place ultraviolet lights in room and bring cord outside of door. Turn on lights for 45 minutes. CAUTION: Do not enter room when UV lights are on.

5. Hang *caution—do not enter* signs on doors leading into area.
6. *After 45 minutes* return UV lights to utility room on floor.
7. Remove all linen, including *plastic pillow cover,* in red linen bag.
8. Remove cubicle curtains and place in a plastic bag.
9. Remove all trash in red plastic bags, using double bag technique.
10. Wash out trash and linen barrels with germicidal solution and place in utility room.
11. Wipe off hand-washing cart with germicidal solution, empty dispensers, and place in utility room.
12. Clean mirror in rest room with germicidal solution. Wash bathroom tiles and window ledge with germicidal solution.
13. Using abrasive pad and cleanser, clean all porcelain and chrome fixtures in rest room.
14. Apply toilet bowl cleaner to swab and clean inside of toilet bowl.
15. With germicidal cloth clean ledges, front of air-conditioner, telephone, bedside table, overbed table, closet, and blood pressure apparatus on wall.
16. Clean mattress (turn over) and bed frame.
17. Wet mop the floor of rest room and patient area. Remove isolation gown, mask, and gloves; discard in trash.
18. Wash hands thoroughly.
19. Make up bed, using a clean plastic pillow cover.
20. Replenish all dispensers in the room—soap, toilet tissue, and hand towels.

Daily cleaning of isolation

EQUIPMENT:

Germicidal solution
Toilet bowl swab
Small bucket
Large bucket
Clean rags
Mop

PROCEDURE:

1. Before entering room, put on isolation gown and gloves. Mask may be optional, depending on the type of isolation. Be sure and check sign outside of door.
2. Clean the bathroom first. Wash all bathroom fixtures, using germicidal solution and clean cloth.
3. Wash all window ledges, blood pressure apparatus on wall, patient furniture, and hand-washing cart with clean cloth and germicidal solution.
4. Replace all needed supplies (toilet paper, paper towels, liquid soap, and hand-washing cart supplies).
5. Mop bathroom and then patient area.
6. All cleaning items taken into the room must be wiped off with a germicidal cloth before they are removed from the room.

7. Empty all wastecans into large trash barrel. Replace plastic lining in wastecan.
8. Trash from large barrels must be double bagged before removing from room. Put new clean red plastic lining in barrel.
9. All rags and mopheads used in the cleaning procedure must be double bagged in a red plastic bag and put on housekeeping cart outside of door.
10. Empty all water. Wipe small bucket and mop bucket with clean germicidal cloth; then place on cart.
11. Remove protective clothing and leave room.

NURSING RESPONSIBILITIES

1. Empty all barrels at end of shift, using double bag technique.
2. Empty basin in hand-washing cart at end of shift and as necessary.
3. Check soap and water dispensers on cart to see that they are filled.
4. Dispose of brown bag used for patient's tissues as necessary.
5. Remove patient's tray.
6. Remove all unnecessary pieces of equipment from room.

SUMMARY TABULATION ON INFECTION CONTROL (ISOLATION TECHNIQUES)*

See Fig. 22 for a sample room setup.

Group I: Enteric precautions

1. Private room	Door open.
2. Gowns	Must be worn by all persons having direct contact with patient.
3. Masks	Not necessary.
4. Hands	*Must* be washed on entering and on leaving room.
5. Gloves	Must be worn by all persons having direct contact

*Based on Public Health Service publications.

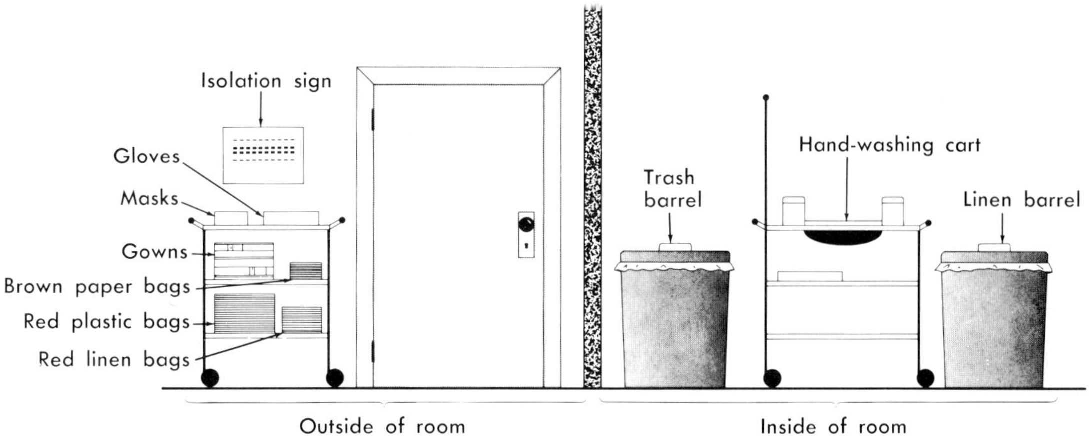

Fig. 22. Room setup.

	with patient or with articles contaminated with fecal material.
6. Articles	Must be double bagged in red plastic bags before removing from room and sending to central service.
7. Linen	Should be placed in trash barrel lined with red linen bag. Must be double bagged in a red linen bag before removing from room and sending to laundry.
8. Trash	Must be double bagged in red plastic bags before removing from room and placing in utility room.
9. Food	An isolation tray must be ordered.
10. Laboratory specimens	Should be double bagged in plastic bags.
11. Transporting the patient	No special precautions are needed unless the patient is incontinent. If the patient is incontinent, he should not be moved from the isolation room.
12. Visitors	Should be instructed on the precautions.

Group II: Wound and skin precautions

1. Private room	Door open.
2. Gowns	Must be worn by all persons having direct contact with patient.
3. Masks	*Not* necessary *except* during dressing changes.
4. Hands	*Must* be washed on entering and leaving room.
5. Gloves	Must be worn by all persons having direct contact with *infected* area.
6. Articles	If the item has come in direct contact with the *infected* area, it should be double bagged in red plastic bags before sending to central service.
7. Linen	Should be placed in trash barrel lined with red linen bag. Must be double bagged in a red linen bag before removing from room and sending to laundry.
8. Trash	Must be double bagged in red plastic bags before removing from room and placing in utility room.
9. Food	No special precautions.
10. Laboratory specimens	No special precautions.
11. Transporting the patient	The infected area should be covered with a sterile barrier towel.
12. Visitors	Should be instructed on the precautions.

Group III: Respiratory isolation

1. Private room	Door open.
2. Gowns	Not necessary.
3. Masks	*Not* needed *unless* patient is unable to cover mouth when coughing or sneezing.
4. Hands	Must be washed on entering and on leaving room.

5. Gloves	Not necessary.
6. Articles	Those contaminated with secretions should be double bagged in a red plastic bag and sent to central service.
7. Linen	No special precautions.
8. Trash	Must be double bagged in red plastic bags before removing from room and placing in utility room.
9. Food	No special precautions.
10. Laboratory specimens	No special precautions.
11. Transporting the patient	The patient should wear a disposable mask when out of the room.
12. Visitors	The patient should wear a mask when visitors are present.

Group IV: Strict isolation

1. Private room	Door must be kept closed.
2. Gowns	Must be worn by all persons entering patient's room.
3. Masks	Must be worn by all persons entering patient's room.
4. Hands	Must be washed on entering and on leaving room.
5. Gloves	Must be worn by all persons entering patient's room.
6. Articles	Must be discarded or double bagged in red plastic bags before being sent to central service.
7. Linen	Should be placed in trash barrel lined with red linen bag. Must be double bagged in a red linen bag before removing from room and sending to laundry.
8. Trash	Must be double bagged in red plastic bags before removing from room and placing in utility room.
9. Food	An isolation tray must be ordered.
10. Laboratory specimens	Should be double bagged in plastic bags.
11. Transporting the patient	The patient should wear an isolation gown as well as mask and gloves. A clean cotton blanket should be placed over the stretcher or wheelchair and then wrapped around the patient.
12. Visitors	Should be limited to two at a time. Before entering room, visitors should be instructed in the use of gowns, masks, and gloves.

Group V: Protective isolation

1. Private room	Door must be kept closed.
2. Gowns	Must be worn by all persons entering room.
3. Masks	Must be worn by all persons entering room.
4. Hands	Must be washed on entering and on leaving room.
5. Gloves	Must be worn by all persons having direct contact with patient.
6. Articles	No special precautions.

7. Linen	Check with physician to see if sterile linens are necessary.
8. Trash	No special precautions.
9. Food	Regular tray may be used.
10. Laboratory specimens	No special precautions.
11. Transporting the patient	Should be curtailed to avoid exposure to any source of infection.
12. Visitors	Visitors should be instructed in the use of gowns, masks and gloves.

Measurement of fluid intake

Container	*Number of milliliters normally given*	*Maximum number of milliliters container holds*
Ice cream carton	120	120
Sherbet carton	120	120
Juice glass (clear plastic)	110	120
Milk glass (clear plastic)	110	120
Milk carton	240	240
Coffee cup (plastic)	150	200
Thermos	250	250
Soup container (plastic)	120	250
Hot cup (styrofoam), small	180	200
Hot cup (styrofoam), large	350	370
Coke bottle (10 oz.)	300	300
7-Up bottle (10 oz.)	300	300
Jello	100	120
Orange juice container (plastic)	120	-
Plastic glass (white)	150	180
Plastic glass (blue)	200	250
Restricted fluids	Amounts marked on containers by dietary	

1 oz. fluid = 30 ml. = 1 medicine cup.
1 oz. ice = 20 ml.

Medication record and narcotic count sheet (Figs. 23 and 24)

PURPOSE: To provide an accurate and complete record of all medications administered to a patient by nursing personnel and physicians.

PROCEDURE:

1. First column is used for list of medications.
   a. Print or write legibly the name, dose, and route of administration—one medication per line.
   b. If the medication is injected (IM or SC), indicate on the line immediately following the medication by writing the word "site."
   c. If medication requires a pulse rate, indicate the type of pulse on the line immediately following the medication (examples, radial, apical).
2. Next five columns.
   a. Date each column with month, day, and year (examples, 1/20/73, 1/21/73, 1/22/73, etc.).

MEDICATION RECORD

Name

Name-Dose-Route	DATE	5/24/73	5/25/73	5/26/73	5/27/73	5/28/73
Lasix 40 mgm iv Push		3P	9A DC			
Keflin Gm 2 iv piggyback		7P	1A-7A-1P-7P	1A-7A-1P-7P	1A-7A DC	
Darvon Cpd. 65 mgm PO		5P				
Digitoxin 0.1 mg PO			9A	(9A)	9A	DC
Record insulin on diabetic record						

Signature of nurse giving team medications	7:30-3:30	P. Green RN	P. Green RN	P. Green RN	P. Green RN	
	3:30-11:30	J. Small RN	J. Small RN	J. Small RN	J. Small RN	
	11:30-7:30		M. Phillips RN	D. Sayer RN	M. Phillips RN	
Signature of nurse giving single PRN medication	7:30-3:30					
	3:30-11:30	S. Brown RN.				
	11:30-7:30					

Fig. 23

b. Under appropriate date, specify hour and indicate whether A.M. or P.M. (examples, 7^A, 11^A, 4^P, 9^P).

c. Chart injection site or pulse rate on line directly under specific time.

d. If both are applicable, use a slash mark and chart in same line space (example, 80/LVG).

e. Medications given between and including times 11:30 P.M. to 7:30 A.M. are charted in *red* ink.

FLOOR: NARCOTIC COUNT SHEET

DATE:															
	7AM	3PM	11P	7AM	3PM	11P	7AM	3PM	11P	7AM	3PM	11P	7AM	3PM	11P
MEPERIDINE 25 mg.															
MEPERIDINE 50 mg.															
MEPERIDINE 50 mg.															
MEPERIDINE 75 mg.															
MEPERIDINE 75 mg.															
MEPERIDINE 100 mg.															
MORPHINE S. 1/6 gr.															
MORPHINE S. 1/8 gr.															
MORPHINE S. 1/4 gr.															
CODEINE 30 mg. Tubex															
CODEINE 60 mg. Tubex															
CODEINE 1/4 gr. tabs															
SECOBARBITAL 3/4 gr.															
SECOBARBITAL 1-1/2gr.															
PENTOBARBITAL 1-1/2gr.															
PHENOBARBITAL amps 2 gr.															
CHLORAL HYDRATE CAPS															
(PAREGORIC) OPIUM CAMPHORATED TINCTURE															
PENTOBARBITAL INJ.															
SECOBARBITAL INJ.															
SIGNATURES (2)															
COMMENTS:															

Fig. 24

3. Signature section at bottom of form.
   a. Team medications—nurse giving *all* medications to that patient for the prescribed 8-hour shift signs record.
   b. p.r.n. medication—a nurse *not assigned to the patient* may give a single p.r.n. or stat medication to the patient. *All* p.r.n. and stat medications require a corresponding note on the nursing record.

   c. Sign in appropriate space according to date, shift, and assignment.
   d. Shift responsibilities for medications are as follows:

      DAY 7:30^{A}-3:30^{P} includes 3:30^{P} medications
      EVENING 3:30^{P}-11:30^{P} includes 11:30^{P} medications
      NIGHT 11:30^{P}-7:30^{A} includes 7:30^{A} medications

4. Withheld medications.
   a. Chart and encircle time (example, 7^{A}).
   b. Record reason in the nurses' notes.
5. Injection site charting—use appropriate sites for IM and SC medications as described on pp. 112 to 117 (anatomical sites of injections and abbreviations).
6. Medications given by physicians (examples, chemotherapy, heparin).
   a. Chart medication completely, as just described.
   b. Write a corresponding note on the nursing record. Include the physician's name.
7. Medications given too frequently for all the times to be charted in one space.
   a. Record as many times as possible in the first space used.
   b. Record additional times in the line space directly below the first space used.
8. Change of dosage or route.
   a. Write DC after final dose.
   b. Rewrite medication, specifying new dose and/or route.
9. Insulin—record on the diabetic control record.
10. Students (professional or licensed practical nurse) who give medications under the supervision of their nursing instructor are to chart the medication, dosage, route, and time but not add their signature. They are to write a corresponding nursing note indicating which medications were given and sign their name.

    EXAMPLE: 1/24/73, 9:00^{A}. All 9:00^{A} P.O. and I.M. medications given.
    Jane Smith, S.N.

11. Drugs (B.S.P. dye, histamine, etc.) used for tests and procedures must be charted by the nurse on the medication sheet, and a corresponding nursing note indicating which physician did the test should be written.

Parenteral hyperalimentation or casein hydrolysate administration

PURPOSE: To administer amino acids, glucose, vitamins, and electrolytes as adequate nutrition for those patients unable to obtain them through the usual digestive route.

POLICY:

Compatibility of drugs: The Pharmacy and Therapeutic Committee has approved that only sodium chloride, potassium chloride, magnesium sulfate, and vitamins be added to hyperalimentation solutions. If any drugs are ordered by the physician to be added, the pharmacy is to notify the physician of the risk involved.

PROCEDURE:

1. The pharmacy will mix the hyperalimentation solution as ordered by the physician.
2. The physician will insert the IV catheter in subclavian vein.
3. The professional nurse will hang the bottle of IV fluids and titrate for a constant rate over 24 hours.
   a. Time tape IV bottle.
   b. Mark IV card with prescribed rate.
   c. Chart on parenteral therapy sheet.
4. The professional nurse will change the IV tubing whenever a new bottle of fluids is hung.
5. The IV catheter site will be cleansed with povidone-iodine, ointment will be applied, and the dressing will be changed every 48 hours by the professional nurse. The dates and time for the dressing change will be noted on the Kardex in the treatment section.
6. The professional nurse will label the date and time of the dressing change and her name on a piece of tape and apply this to the outside of the dressing. This should be done when she changes the dressing.
7. The kind and amounts of IV fluids that are hung and are infused will be noted on the bedside I & O graphic by the professional nurse or her designate.
8. The following treatments are usually indicated for patients receiving hyperalimentation fluids. These treatments should be ordered by the physician and carried out by the nurse.
   a. Record a strict I & O.
   b. Weigh the patient daily.
   c. Do spot-check urine on a double-voided urine specimen at least every 6 hours as ordered by the physician; patient will usually be covered by sliding scale for insulin.

POTENTIAL COMPLICATIONS AND PREVENTION:

A. Sepsis
   1. Hyperalimentation solution provides an excellent environment for bacterial, yeast, and fungal growth. The nurse can help prevent contamination by the following means:
      a. Administering the solution as soon after mixing as possible.
      b. Placing the bottles in the refrigerator if the solution is not administered immediately.
      c. Using only unopened bottles in which a vacuum is present and using new IV tubing for each bottle of fluids.
      d. Inspecting the solution and bottle before patient administration and also during the administration to ensure that it is absolutely clear and free of any particulate matter, haze, or cloudiness; the container should be inspected for any physical damage such as cracks.
      e. Discarding the unused contents of a bottle when administration is discontinued.

f. *Never*
  (1) Let a bottle hang longer than prescribed time (usually 8 hours).
  (2) Give medications or blood through the hyperalimentation line.
  (3) Do a C.V.P. through the hyperalimentation line.
  (4) Break the hyperalimentation line except for changing bottles or in an emergency.
  (5) Draw blood through the hyperalimentation line.

2. The entrance of microorganisms around the catheter site can be prevented by
   a. The physician using aseptic technique when inserting the catheter.
   b. Cleansing the catheter insertion site and applying a sterile dressing every 48 hours, using sterile technique.

B. Hyperglycemia, glycosuria, and osmotic dehydration may result from excessive administration of glucose, as shown by the symptoms listed. The nurse may help in the following ways:
   1. Never increase the IV rate to compensate for any interruption or slowing.
   2. Never administer at a rate greater than 1 liter in 3 hours.
   3. Minimize by slowing the infusion rate.

   Symptoms of too rapid infusion

   Early: Headache, nausea, increased lassitude, flushing of skin.
   Late: Glycosuria, osmotic diuresis, dehydration, coma, convulsions.

Parenteral therapy record and Flo-Meter indicator tapes (Figs. 25 and 26)

PURPOSE: To provide a method of controlling the administration of intravenous solutions, including their labeling and recording.

EQUIPMENT:

Parenteral therapy record.
Flo-Meter indicator tape (1000 ml. or 500 ml.).
Intravenous solution as ordered.

PROCEDURE:

A. To *label solution*
   1. Select the appropriate Flo-Meter tape.
   2. Fill in the information as follows:
      a. Solution: Amount and type.
      b. Bottle number: Must correspond with the bottle number (or letter) on the IV card.
      c. Patient: Full name.
      d. Room no.: Include bed number.
      e. Med. added: Name and dose or write "none."
      f. Date: Day, month, year when IV bottle is started.
      g. Starting time: Specify hour and whether A.M. or P.M. (examples, 7^{A}, 3^{P}).
      h. Drops per minute: Calculated rate. Milliliter per hour rate or "KVO" may be written in the empty box next to the drops per minute box.

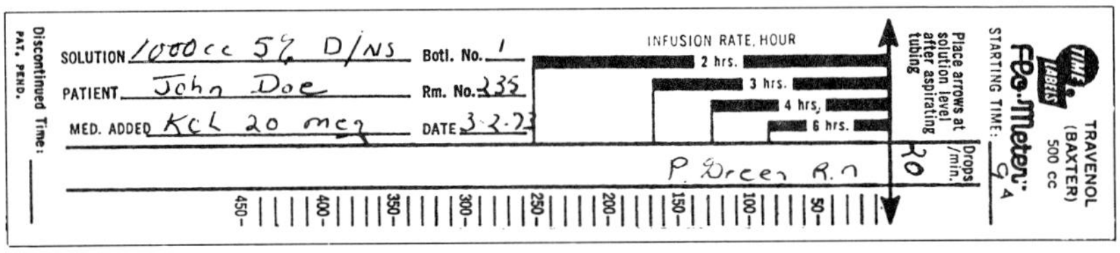

Fig. 25

Flo-Meter

In-Service Guide for Viaflex container

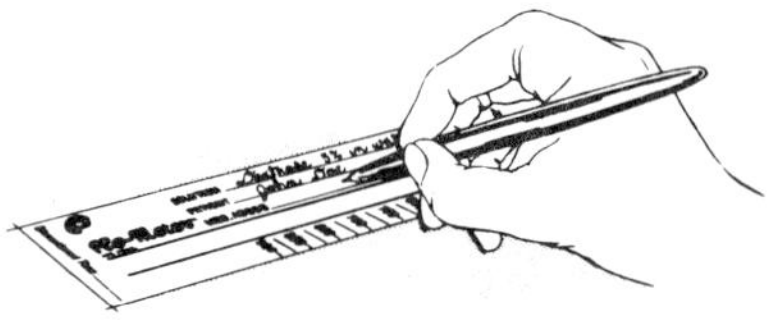

1 Determine the prescribed rate: drops/minute or ml/hr. Fill in the patient information and indicate medication added, if any, in the space alloted.

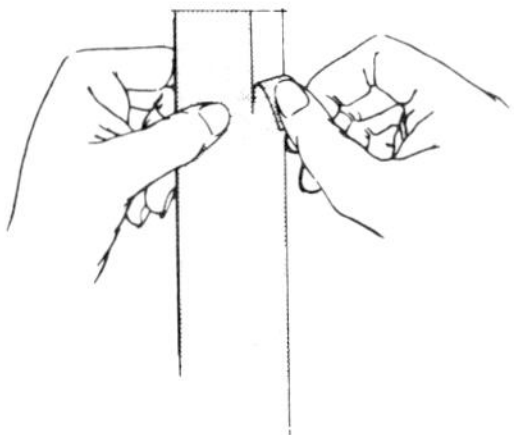

2 Remove only narrow strip of the backing paper before applying to Viaflex container.

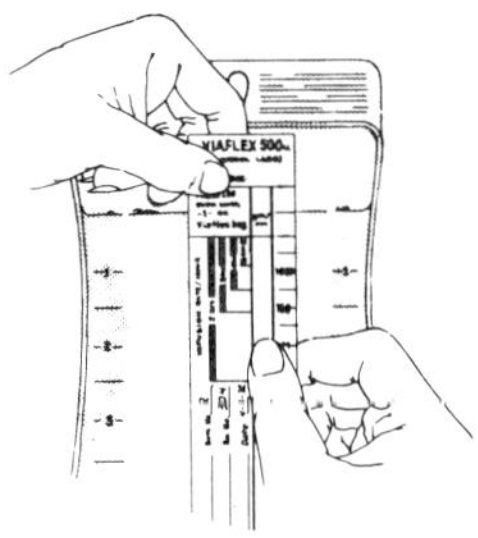

3 Apply label to the Viaflex container with 100 ▶ on label at same level as – 1 – on the Viaflex container.

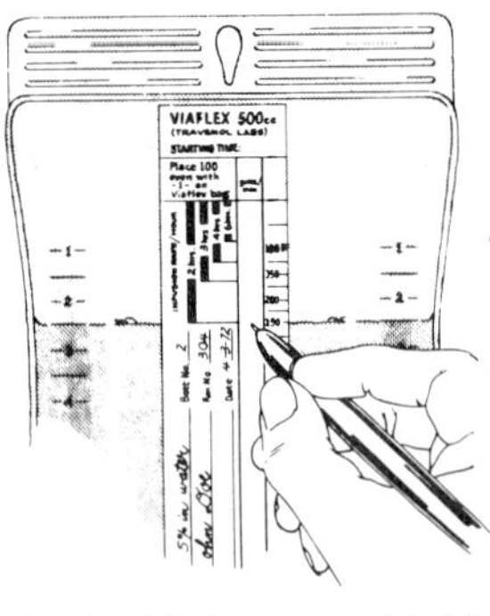

4

First hour rate of Infusion may be checked by volume chart. Recording in pen or pencil can be made directly on label.

5 After infusion, remove label from Viaflex container and remove remaining backing paper. Label can now be placed into patient's permanent record.

Additional infusions will require a new Flo-meter label.

TIME PRODUCTS — PROFESSIONAL TAPE COMPANY, INC.
144 TOWER DRIVE, BURR RIDGE (HINSDALE), ILLINOIS 60521

Fig. 26

i. The R.N. preparing IV must sign first initial, last name, and R.N. in space just below the "Drops/min." box.

NOTE: When bottle is smaller than 500 ml., fill in the Flo-Meter tape as directed in points a through i. Draw line through nonapplicable cc. numbers on the ruler-like section.

B. To *apply* Flo-Meter tape to solution
   1. Remove only the *narrow* strip of backing.
   2. Invert IV bottle, align arrows on tape with fluid level, then affix tape.
   3. Do this *after* medication has been added and tubing aspirated.
   4. Use a paper clip to attach tape to blood or plasma bag.

C. To *end* the solution
   1. Remove the label from the bottle and remove the remaining backing paper.
   2. Place the label in the next open space on the parenteral therapy record. Do *not* skip spaces. When front side of record is filled, use back side.
   3. Person removing the tape must
      a. Write the "discontinued time" in the appropriate space.
      b. Sign name and status just above this time.
      c. Write the total number of cc. absorbed.
      d. Add "Dc'd" if IV infusion is terminated.

NOTE: When patient has continuous IV fluid infusions, the following routine must be followed:
   1. Change all IV tubing every 24 hours.
   2. Change all site dressings and apply antiseptic ointment every 24 hours.
   3. Indicate time on treatment section of the Kardex when IV tubing and site dressing are to be changed every day.
   4. *No* IV bottle is to infuse for longer than 24 hours.

Parenteral therapy record (Fig. 27)

PURPOSE: To provide a continuous and complete record of all parenteral solutions administered to a patient.

PROCEDURE:
   1. Chart *all* parenteral fluids on this form, including blood, platelets, and albumin.
   2. *All information must be complete.*
   3. Bottle number must correspond with the IV card in the Kardex. All fluids must be numbered or lettered to avoid confusion.
   4. Chart the solution as mixed, including all medications added.
      a. "Started" and "Solution" sections must be completed immediately on hanging any bottle or bag.
      b. "Completed" section must be filled in immediately by the person removing fluid bottle or bag.

Peritoneal dialysis

PURPOSE: A technique for removing excessive body wastes, excessive body fluid, excessive serum electrolytes, and toxic ingestions.

PARENTERAL THERAPY RECORD

J. Doe 405'

STARTED				SOLUTION	COMPLETED				
Date	Time	Signature	Bottle Number	Amount-Type-Medications	Date	Time	Amount Absorbed	Signature	Comments
1-20-72	9^{A}	P. Green RN	# 1	1000 cc 5% D/LR c̄ 40 Meq KCL	1-20-72	5^{P}	1000 cc	R. Reed R.N.	
1-20-72	5P	R. Reed RN	# 2	1000 cc N Saline c̄ Solu B&C. Amp. i	1-21-72	1a	1000 cc	M. Blue RN.	
				and 20 meq K.C.L.					
1-21-72	1 A	M. Blue	# 3	500 cc 5% D/W	1-21-72	5^{30} A	200 cc	M. Blue	Infiltrated
1-21-72	8^{30} A	P. Green	# 1	1000 cc N.S	1-21-72	3P	800 cc	P. Green	discontinued
1-21-72	5p	R. Red RN	# 2	500 cc whole blood	1-21-72	7P	500 cc	R. Red RN	

Fig. 27

POINTS OF EMPHASIS:

1. A signed operative permit must be obtained from the patient.
2. Strict aseptic technique is to be used when the physician inserts the catheter into peritoneal cavity.
3. The professional nurse is to use sterile technique when adding medications to the dialysate fluid and in hanging the fluids.
4. The following medications can be added to the dialysate per order of the physician.
   a. Heparin—to minimize the fibrinous deposits on the catheter, which may impede the exchange of fluid.
   b. Antibiotics—to decrease the possibility of peritonitis.
   c. Potassium—when serum potassium is normal or below normal, it is customary to add potassium.
5. If the patient experiences severe pain during the exchange, the physician might order procaine.

6. The initial outflow drainage may be pink tinged, but this should disappear after several cycles. If bleeding continues, notify the physician.
7. The drainage is usually straw colored.
8. If leakage occurs around the catheter or if the drainage becomes slow or erratic, notify the physician.
9. The patient should be observed for
   a. Respiratory difficulty
   b. Severe abdominal pain
   c. Bleeding
   d. Shock
   e. Leakage

   If any of the above conditions occur, notify the physician.
10. Cycle length—usually one cycle will take from 40 minutes to a little over an hour.
    a. 5 to 10 minutes for the fluid to flow in.
    b. 30 to 45 minutes for the fluid to remain in the peritoneal cavity.
    c. 10 to 20 minutes for the fluid to drain out.

    Usually 30 to 40 cycles will be exchanged.
11. It is common to get an incomplete return with the first few exchanges.
12. The patients may be turned without harm during the procedure. Repositioning the patient on his side during the procedure is necessary to maintain skin integrity and promote comfort. It may also increase the flow of the drainage when this does not flow in a steady stream or drips very slowly.
13. Gentle massage of the abdomen may also increase the output of fluid.
14. A 7% dextrose solution may be used for removal of excessive body fluid. There are the following risks when using a 7% solution: acute pulmonary edema, hypovolemia, and shock. Rarely should more than 2 or 3 such exchanges be done.
15. Be sure the outflow clamp is off before allowing solution to run.

PROCEDURE:

1. Operative permit should be obtained.
2. The dialysis fluid is obtained from the pharmacy as ordered by the physician and the peritoneal dialysis tray and tubing are obtained from central service.
3. Patient should be weighed.
4. Additional equipment you might have at the bedside—tape, 4 × 4's, povidone-iodine swabs, tincture of benzoin.
5. Take patient's temperature, pulse, respiration, and blood pressure prior to the dialysis.
6. Have patient empty his bladder.
7. Place patient in a supine position.
8. The physician will shave and drape the patient's abdomen. Using sterile technique, he will insert a trocar into the peritoneum. A catheter will be inserted through the trocar and positioned. A purse-string suture is looped around the catheter. A sterile dressing is placed around the catheter.

9. A Y-tubing is connected to the catheter and 2 liters of warmed dialysate should run in rapidly by gravity. (Warm the dialysate in a pan of warm water; solution should be at body temperature to prevent abdominal distress.)
10. Note the times on the flow sheet that the bottles were allowed to drain, as well as when they became completely empty.
11. Take patient's vital signs every 15 minutes during the first cycle and then every hour.

PERITONEAL DIALYSIS FLOWSHEET

Key: Fluid and cumulative balance

- means excess peritoneal fluid expelled
+ means fluid retained in peritoneal cavity

PREDIALYSIS WT.________ POSTDIALYSIS WT.________

DATE	TIMES	DIALYSIS CYCLE NUMBER	TYPE SOLUTION WITH MEDICATIONS	VOLUME		FLUID BALANCE	FLUID CUMULATIVE BALANCE	REMARKS AND SIGNATURES
				IN	OUT			

Fig. 28

12. Take patient's temperature every 4 hours.
13. Allow fluid to remain in peritoneal cavity for the prescribed period of time—30 to 45 minutes.
14. The fluid is then drained by a siphon effect through a closed system. If the system is patent, gravity drainage should occur rapidly and a steady stream of fluid should be seen entering the drainage container.
15. Just before the drainage is initiated, more dialysate fluid is prepared and set up so that as soon as drainage ceases, a new infusion can be started.
16. The drainage should be accurately measured and recorded on the flow sheet.
17. The procedure is repeated continuously for as many cycles as the physician orders.
18. The *peritoneal dialysis flow sheet* (Fig. 28) must be completed for each cycle.

Physician's order sheet (Fig. 29)

The order sheet will contain three copies: (1) copy (original) for the patient's permanent record, (2) copy for pharmacy departmental file, and (3) copy for the business office.

The order sheet is 11 × 8½ inches and consists of an original sheet with two copies. Each sheet has three large detachable sections for writing orders. At the bottom of each section a place is allotted for the physician's signature and BNDD number, also for the nurse's signature. Each detachable section of the sheet is numbered and can be used for tracing the physician's orders.

METHODOLOGY

Before the order sheet is inserted in the order book, the patient's name must be imprinted on the three sections of the sheet.

The physician should write firmly with a ball-point pen. Medication orders should be written clearly and include the name of the drug, dosage, directions, route of administration, and the quantity when necessary.

The general orders are written in the same section of the order sheet, using the same procedure.

The completed orders are signed by the physician, who adds his BNDD number.

The order sheet is ready to be forwarded to the pharmacy after the sheet is checked to see that all pertinent information has been added. The second and third copies of each completed order are removed from the order sheet. These copies are sent to the pharmacy. The first copy is the permanent copy for patient's record.

Stat orders may be telephoned to the pharmacy and a stat dose will be sent; the order sheet may be sent later.

Discharge orders should be marked discharge before the order sheet is sent to the pharmacy.

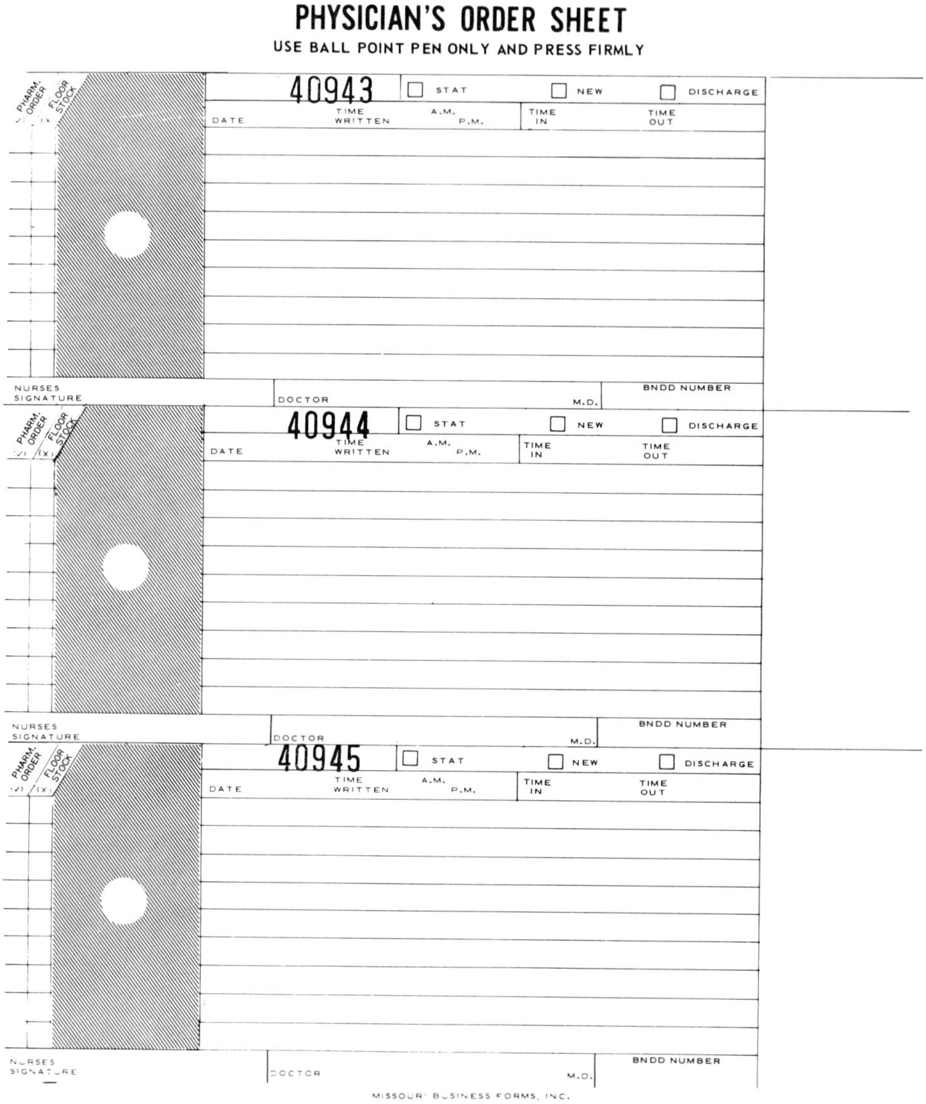

PHYSICIAN'S ORDER SHEET
USE BALL POINT PEN ONLY AND PRESS FIRMLY

PHARM. ORDER (√) | FLOOR STOCK (X) | 40943 | ☐ STAT | ☐ NEW | ☐ DISCHARGE
DATE | TIME WRITTEN | A.M. P.M. | TIME IN | TIME OUT
NURSES SIGNATURE | DOCTOR M.D. | BNDD NUMBER

PHARM. ORDER (√) | FLOOR STOCK (X) | 40944 | ☐ STAT | ☐ NEW | ☐ DISCHARGE
DATE | TIME WRITTEN | A.M. P.M. | TIME IN | TIME OUT
NURSES SIGNATURE | DOCTOR M.D. | BNDD NUMBER

PHARM. ORDER (√) | FLOOR STOCK (X) | 40945 | ☐ STAT | ☐ NEW | ☐ DISCHARGE
DATE | TIME WRITTEN | A.M. P.M. | TIME IN | TIME OUT
NURSES SIGNATURE | DOCTOR M.D. | BNDD NUMBER

MISSOURI BUSINESS FORMS, INC.

Fig. 29

Refill prescriptions should be sent to the pharmacy with the original container and a refill pharmacy requisition. This can continue until the physician discontinues the medication.

Drugs ordered on the order sheet that are floor stock can be used from floor stock supply. The box marked floor stock on the order sheet should be checked, signifying that this item is floor stock. A pharmacy requisition must be written for replacement of all floor stock.

A physician's telephoned orders may be taken by a nurse and written in the order book. The nurse should write the letters T.O. beside her name in the signature. The physician can sign the order on his next visit to the hospital.

PHARMACY PROCEDURE

When the order sheet arrives in the pharmacy, it will be checked by a pharmacist for medication orders. This departmental copy will be used as a prescription number to be stamped on each medication order. This number will be placed on the same line the drug is written on. This same number will be stamped on the prescription label and will contain the patient's name, date, room number, drug, dosage, and name of the physician who ordered the medication.

All control drugs written on the order sheet will be transcribed by a pharmacist to a pharmacy requisition referring to the number on the order sheet. The order sheet contains the physician's BNDD number. The transcribed requisition will contain a prescription, date, patient's name, number of order sheet, room number, drug, quantity, dosage, and the physician's name.

Five days' supply of medication will be sent if the quantity is not specified. All narcotics orders will be filled with a 72-hour supply.

Refill prescriptions will be filled when the prescription is refillable and the container is sent with the refill requisition.

Preoperative checklist (Fig. 30)

PURPOSE: To ensure that the patient is completely prepared for surgery before leaving the nursing unit.

PROCEDURE:

1. The secretary stamps and places the checklist on the front of the patient's chart by 4 P.M. the evening prior to surgery.
2. *"Evening before surgery" section:*
   a. The team leader completes the first part before 7 P.M.
   b. The unit secretary completes the second part before 7 P.M.
   N.B. If this section cannot be completed for any reason, the physician should be notified.
3. *"Day of surgery" section:*
   a. The team leader completes this section, which includes a final check on all items.
   b. The L.P.N. and/or the nursing attendant prepares the patient and then reports to the team leader those items that are completed.
4. Only after the checklist is completed may the patient go to surgery.

Temperature record (Fig. 31)

PURPOSE: To provide a continuous record of temperatures, pulses, respirations, weights, bowel habits, and the 24-hour intake and output summary.

PROCEDURE:

A. Date: Include month, day, and year (example, 1/21/74).

B. Day: May be used for indicating the following:

Adm.—day of admission
2—days after admission
Surg.—day of surgery
1 P.O.—first post-op. day

PRE-OPERATIVE CHECK LIST

Check if Completed

WARD SECRETARY

- ______ Stamps the pre-operative check list, attaches it to the front of the chart and places on the desk
- ______ Notifies the Chaplain and checks the chart for the following and notifies the appropriate person if any of the items are not done
- ______ History and physical
- ______ Consultations
- ______ Physician's orders signed
- ______ Pre-operative orders signed
- ______ Chest x-ray report obtained
- ______ EKG report obtained
- ______ CBC report obtained
- ______ Urinalysis report obtained
- ______ Type and cross match done
  No. of units of blood available______

Signature:______________________

UNIT MANAGER

- ______ ID band on
- ______ Jewelry and other valuables removed and secured
- ______ Notify family

Signature:______________________

TEAM LEADER

- ______ Operative permit obtained. If not obtained by 7 p.m., notify the appropriate resident. If permit is still not obtained, notify attending M.D. and O.R.
- ______ NPO after midnight placed on bed

Signature:______________________

DAY OF SURGERY

TEAM LEADER

- ______ Bath, mouth care, gown
- ______ TPR, BP, and weight recorded
- ______ Contact lense, glasses, dentures removed and given to Unit Manager
- ______ Voided at ____ amount ________
- ______ Pre-op drugs given and charted
- ______ Nurses' notes signed off
- ______ I & O and Parenteral Therapy Sheet from clip board to chart
- ______ Drug order sheet in chart
- ______ Pre-op check list - final check

Signature:______________________

Fig. 30

C. Temperature:
   1. Chart by darkening the appropriate dot next to the correct temperature and under the correct time.
   2. Rectal temperatures are designated by a capital letter R immediately above the dot.
   3. Axillary temperatures are designated by a capital letter A immediately above the dot.

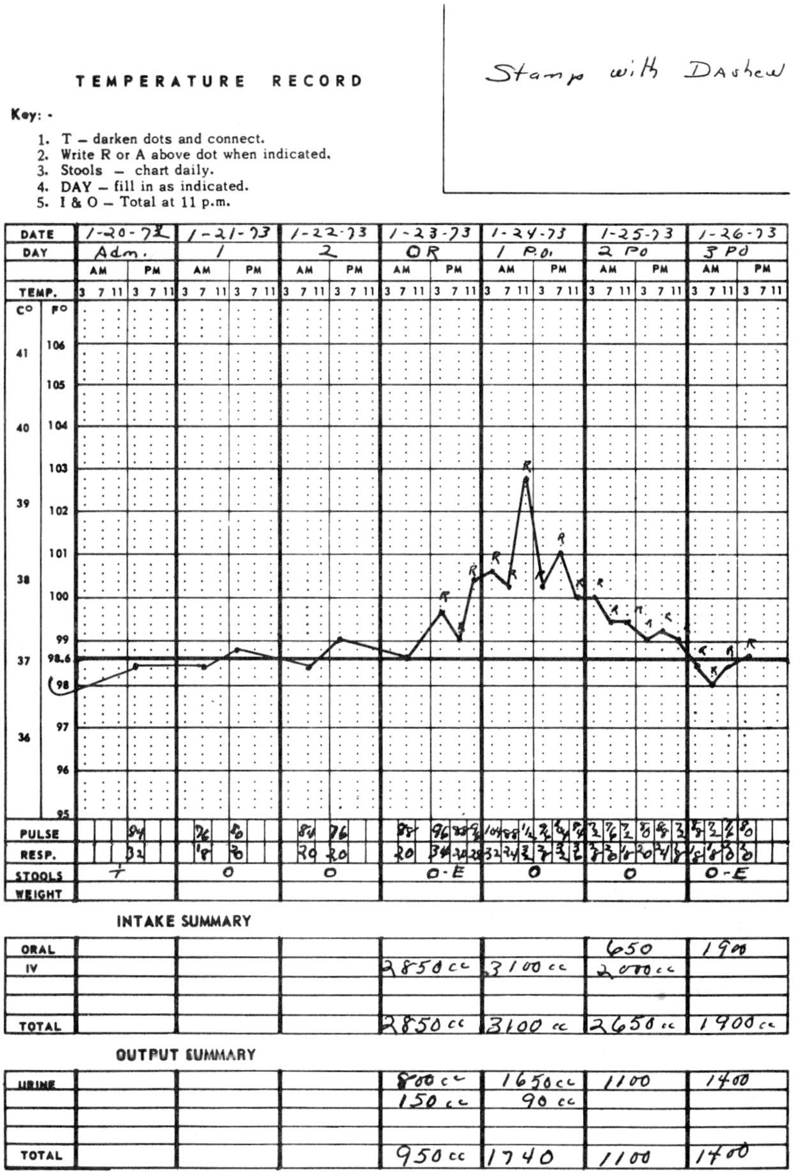

Fig. 31

D. Pulse and respirations: Write vertically in the designated space under the correct time.

EXAMPLE:

Pulse	108	84
Resp.	32	24

E. Stools:
   1. Chart daily, using the following symbols:

      $\bar{i}$ = Yes   0 = No   E = Enema

   2. Chart frequency (examples, 2 ×, 3 ×, E × 3).
   3. Observations of unusual signs (color, consistency, odor, etc.) must be recorded in the nurses' notes.
   4. Results of enemas must be recorded in the nurses' notes.

F. Weight: Write beneath the correct date and indicate whether weight is in kilograms (kg.) or in pounds (lb.).

G. Intake and output summary:
   1. The 11-7:30 shift is responsible for
      a. Collecting
      b. Totaling
      c. Recording
      d. Placing new sheet on clipboard

      } done at 11 P.M.
   2. Chart the totals beneath the date of the current day. Example: At 11 P.M., 1/21/74, chart the totals from the previous 24 hours under 1/21/74. This date (1/21/74) corresponds with the date on the I & O sheet from which the totals have been obtained.
   3. When recording, use the blank spaces for fluids other than those indicated on the sheet.

Tracheostomy care

PURPOSE: A surgical incision into the trachea for the insertion of a tube to provide a patent airway and to facilitate the removal of excess bronchial secretions.

The cuffed tube is used most frequently (1) in combination with a positive pressure aspirator for the patient who requires mechanical assistance in ventilation and (2) to reduce the chances of aspiration in patients whose laryngeal and pharyngeal protective reflexes are lost.

DESCRIPTIONS: A tracheostomy tube is a plastic or metal curved tube about 2½ to 4 inches long, which fits in and downward into the tracheal opening. The tube consists of an outer cannula to which are attached tapes that tie around the patient's neck so that hard coughing will not eject the tube. An inner cannula (although not all tubes have an inner cannula) fits inside the outer cannula and fastens. The third part is the obturator—a plug that is placed inside and extends through the outer cannula to provide a blunt point when the trach tube is inserted into the trachea. This is removed and replaced by the inner cannula as soon as the tracheostomy tube is in position. The obturator must be taped to the head of the bed, in full view, for use in case the tube needs to be reinserted in cases of emergencies.

The cuff, usually made of soft rubber, encircles the lower portion of the outer cannula of the tracheostomy tube. Once the tube is in place in the patient's trachea, the cuff is inflated to form a seal between the tracheostomy tube and the trachea. The only route for effective air exchange, with the cuff inflated, is the lumen of the tracheostomy tube. The inflated cuff also reduces the possibility of aspiration of secretions into the lower trachea and bronchi. The cuff is inflated by injecting air into the fine-bore tubing that leads to the cuff. The small pilot balloon located near the distal end of the tubing acts as an indicator of whether or not the cuff is inflated. The end of the tubing may or may not be flanged to fit a syringe tip. Some models have a self-sealing valve at the end of the tubing.

TYPES OF TUBES AVAILABLE:

1. Jackson trachea tube—metal tube that comes in sizes 5 through 8, in short or long. These may be ordered with or without an inflatable cuff.
2. Kistner tube—tube that consists of two parts: cannula and cap. These are made of green plastic. There is no inner cannula or obturator.
3. Portex tube—tube that has inflatable cuff and has no inner cannula.
4. The Schweiss tube—metal tube that has a self-inflating cuff. These come in sizes 7 or 8, short or long. (Obtained from O.R.)
5. Shiley trach tube—disposable trach tube with a low pressure cuff, coming in sizes 4, 6, 8, 10.
6. Lanz trach tube—disposable trach tube with a controlled pressure cuff. There is no inner cannula or obturator. Lanz tubes come in sizes 6 through 10.

POLICY:

1. A tracheostomy is done in the operating room except in cases of emergency when there is not enough time to move the patient to the O.R.
2. A tracheostomy tray is kept on the emergency cart on each nursing division.
3. A duplicate sterile tracheostomy tube must be kept at the bedside.
4. A hemostat must be taped to the top of the bed.
5. The obturator must be taped to the top of the bed.
6. Specific orders should be written by the physician and indicate each of the following:
   a. Amount of air used for cuff inflation
   b. Frequency and duration of cuff deflation
   c. Type of humidification
   d. If the cuff should be inflated before feeding
7. Anyone suctioning a trach or doing tracheostomy care must wear a mask and sterile gloves.

COMPLICATIONS: Three serious complications to guard against are suffocation, aspiration, and tracheal ischemia.

PRECAUTIONS AND POINTS OF EMPHASIS:

1. Never remove the outer cannula. It is to be changed only by the doctor. The inner cannula may be removed for cleaning.
2. If the patient shows signs of cyanosis or difficulty in breathing or if the tube becomes dislocated, call the doctor at once. If the outer cannula is expelled, keep the airway open with a hemostat.

3. Frank blood, obtained later than the immediate postoperative period, must be reported. (Postoperatively, bloody mucus is normal.)
4. Always use aseptic technique in changing the tracheostomy dressing, in cleaning the inner cannula, and in suctioning.
5. Do not use cotton-filled dressings or cotton applicators around a tracheostomy.
6. All tracheostomy patients have some tracheobronchial secretions. Report if no secretions can be aspirated. This may indicate inadequate humidification.
7. Inspired air should be continuously and adequately humidified. This is the most important factor in preventing the formation of crusts.
8. Keep the nebulizer tubing below the level of the trachea. This permits condensation to drain back into the reservoir and prevents it from running into the trachea.
9. The cuff should be deflated when the respirator is not in use unless inflation is specifically ordered by the physician.
10. Close observation is necessary if the patient is being ventilated with a respirator, since a mechanical failure could result in asphyxiation.
11. Do not overinflate the cuff. Inject the least amount of air necessary to adequately inflate the cuff and seal the trachea. An alert patient may complain of a sensation of tightness or choking if the cuff is overinflated.
12. Hourly deflation of the cuff for 3 to 5 minutes is necessary, to prevent tracheal ischemia.
13. Never deflate the cuff until the oronasal pharynx has been suctioned. Pooled secretion above the cuff could be released to flood the bronchi.
14. Be sure the airway is patent when reinflating the cuff. A weakness in the rubber occasionally allows a ballooning of the cuff over the end of the tracheostomy tube, thus occluding it.
15. Notify the physician immediately if there is any difficulty in inflating the cuff. A cuff leak or rupture will require replacement of the tube by the physician. The cuff may be defective if (a) the pilot balloon does not remain inflated after the clamp is applied; (b) the air from the syringe enters the fine-bore tubing with no resistance, and large amounts of air do not seal the area between the tube and the trachea; (c) more air can be withdrawn from the fine-bore tubing than was originally injected; (d) the patient continues to be able to speak; and (e) the positive pressure respirator triggers continuously or fails to maintain the system pressure as set by the control pressure.
16. Provide tools for the patient's communication—call bell and magic slate or pad and pencil.
17. Frequent visits to the bedside will help assure the patient that help is near and that the equipment is operating satisfactorily.

INFLATING THE CUFF:

1. Fill the syringe with 8 to 10 cc. of air (as ordered).
2. Connect the respirator.
3. Insert syringe into the self-sealing valve or flanged end of tubing (if not flanged, insert a 16-gauge blunt needle into end of tubing). Inject a small amount of air until there is no audible hissing of escaping air around the tube.

Draw back again on the syringe until there is the slightest of leaks and then inject a slight amount more to seal the trachea.

4. Using the flat clip provided with the set, clamp the cuff tubing off, between the pilot balloon and the distal end. Remove the syringe. The small pilot balloon should now be partially inflated.
5. Respirator should cycle efficiently, maintaining the pressure as set by the control pressure.
6. Record the time of inflation and the amount of air used to inflate the cuff on the Kardex as well as in the nurses' notes.

DEFLATING THE CUFF:

1. *Always* suction the oronasal pharynx before deflating the cuff.
2. Remove the clip from the fine-bore tubing to allow the air to escape and the cuff to deflate. Check that the tubing does not stay pinched; the pilot balloon should also deflate.
3. Leave deflated for 3 to 5 minutes if the respirator will operate. Deflation may have to be shortened if the patient is being deprived of oxygen.
4. Record time and duration of deflation on the Kardex as well as the nurses' notes.

EQUIPMENT:

Wall suction or electric suction apparatus

Tracheostomy care set (disposable) for cleaning inner cannula:

- 1 Plastic tray with 2 compartments
- 1 Removable plastic basin
- 1 Pair gloves
- 1 Cleaning brush
- 1 Towel
- 4 Gauze sponges (4 × 4 inch)
- 4 Pipe cleaners (large)
- 2 Swabs
- 2 Twill tapes (½ × 15 inch)
- 1 Tracheostomy dressing
- 1 Large waterproof drape

PROCEDURE:

1. Peel lid from tray.
2. Remove drape and position on patient and work surface.
3. Remove separate blue basin and place contents on sterile field.
4. Fill basins with hydrogen peroxide and normal saline.
5. Put on sterile gloves.
6. Remove inner cannula and place in peroxide solution.
7. Cleanse the inner cannula by using tracheostomy brush or pipe cleaners.
8. Rinse cannula in saline. Drain on a gauze flat.
9. Apply new dressings.
10. Reinsert cannula and fasten; suction patient.
11. Discard tray.
12. Repeat procedure every 4 hours or oftener for a fresh tracheostomy, if necessary, to prevent crust formation.

13. Leave patient comfortable.

Tracheostomy suctioning

PRECAUTIONS AND POINTS OF EMPHASIS:

1. Never use in the trachea a catheter that has been used for suctioning mouth and pharynx.
2. The catheter should be a size smaller than the lumen of the tracheostomy tube (usually no. 14 or 16).
3. Suction should be applied intermittently for periods of no longer than 5 seconds.
4. Do not push the catheter in and out, since this may damage the mucosa.
5. Encourage patients to clear the bronchi by coughing so that suctioning is less traumatic.

EQUIPMENT:

Portable or wall suction apparatus.
Sterile saline (500 ml. bottle).
Suction kit.
  Catheter (14F, 16F, 18F).
  Gloves.
  Disposable cup.
Wastebasket with plastic lining.

PROCEDURE:

1. Wash hands.
2. Open suction kit.
3. Assemble disposable cup on sterile field wrap.
4. Pour normal saline into disposable cup.
5. Put on sterile disposable gloves. (Handle the nonsterile items with the same hand, keeping one glove sterile to handle the suction catheter.)
6. Connect catheter to suction tubing.
7. Lubricate tip with sterile saline solution and, with suction off, gently insert catheter into tracheostomy as far as it will go without pressure. Avoid "poking." Pull catheter back about 1 cm., to free tip from bronchus wall, and apply by placing the thumb over the Regu-Vac of the catheter. Slowly withdraw the catheter while rotating it between the fingers. If the catheter grabs, release the suction by removing thumb from vent.
8. Rinse the catheter with saline solution and repeat the procedure for other main bronchus. (Turn head to right to aspirate left bronchus; to left to aspirate right bronchus.)
9. Continue to suction the patient until he appears free of secretions, allowing time between aspirations for oxygenating the patient.
10. At completion of the procedure, rinse the tubing with saline solution and discard soiled catheter, gloves, and disposable cup.
11. Empty suction bottle at end of shift or sooner if necessary.
12. Check to see there are additional suction kits.

CHAPTER 4

Conclusions and recommendations

REPORT AND OBSERVATIONS

The orientation and evaluation program described in this text was constructed and planned to give the professional nurse both a very detailed concept of her responsibilities and the tools necessary to fulfill those responsibilities with the greatest degree of freedom and a recognition of her contribution to patient welfare in the hospital setting.

Changes must be brought about by a deliberate yet controlled process. Clinical nurses on the staff had for several months complained about the orientation program then in use. Many unfreezing forces had been in action. The design of the changes had been discussed many times with the clinical nurses and they had verbalized their acceptance for change. Regardless, it must be remembered that change cannot take place without some anxiety.

During the first two weeks of orientation we found very few problems. The young graduate had no problem in participating as a team member or, during that period, in administering medications and performing other technical activities.

In the third week of orientation the anxieties of the clinical nurse and the nursing staff began to surface. The clinical nurses expressed concerns and fears that the new graduate would fail her evaluation and thus have her employment terminated. Further, it was feared that she really could not utilize self-directed learning or organize and manage the nursing team. Most of the clinical nurses urged us to go back to the old method of orientation. The L.P.N.s and nurses' aides were quick to pick up the cry, and they too expressed fears and doubts that the new professional could function properly.

This is the period when close observation, counseling, and control must be exercised.

All participants were assured that we did appreciate and understand their concern. They were helped to understand that professional nurses, like members of other professions (doctors, lawyers, engineers, and teachers), experience tension-ridden and anxiety-laden moments during their educational programs and early careers. The majority of young people entering the professions do not judge such experiences as catastrophic. They recognize the pain of conflict but want help on their own terms. They want the right to ask for help when they need it but to have freedom to act in those areas in which they feel confident. All clinical nurses were assured that we did not intend to revert to the old method but would proceed with the program as planned. This stand, or course, was accepted and we heard no more about doubts, fears, or going back to the four-week orientation program formerly in use.

The third week of orientation was marked by absolute quiet from all the units. The units appeared to be functioning with a greater degree of team spirit. The patients seemed to be well cared for and there was no evidence of staff anxiety.

The end result was that team members immediately created an atmosphere in which the various levels of nursing personnel could interact with mutual respect. Everyone made a greater effort to do her best in the most efficient and empathetic way. Staff members were more attentive on walking rounds, participated in team conferences, and showed a greater degree of concern for patient welfare. The new team goal appeared to be one of assisting *their new graduate* in making the highest score with the least possible transitional pain.

During the fourth and fifth weeks the young graduate could be observed conducting walking rounds and team conferences, with self-confidence and understanding.

We have now completed the evaluation of twenty-two graduates. The lowest score made was 78.5 on the competency rating scale and 88 on the nursing care audit. The mean of the group was 86.

It was interesting to note that although the new goal of the team members was one of helping their team leader the end result was improved patient care.

EVALUATIONS BY OTHERS

Clinical nurses

Two of the most experienced of the eleven clinical nurses were asked to give us their evaluation of the program. The first respondent gave the following reply:

> I did not think it would work, but I have been made a believer.

The second described the following:

> When we realized we could not revert to the old method as a result of increased pressure, we vowed among ourselves that our new graduate would not fail. We told all team members to help the new graduate so that she could function and make a high grade on evaluation.

Patients

During their hospitalization, patients showed significant improvement in care. Dissatisfaction with care received, as expressed by evaluation, dropped from 9.4% in May of 1973 to 1.7% in January of 1974.

Newly graduated nurses

One of the most important elements in evaluating a program is the evaluation of those participating in the activity.

During the interviews for employment the program was explained to each individual, and all were informed that we would ask for their evaluation after the six-week experience. They were asked to focus on specific procedures that they felt least prepared to perform or incidents in which they felt frustrated, not knowing how to interact.

The following comments are from the evaluation of twenty-five graduate nurses. The group included seventeen baccalaureate graduates and eight Associate Degree or Diploma Program graduates.

The evaluations of the nurses who were oriented by the described program were reviewed for positive and negative attitudes. The following are comments: One of the respondents related the following:

> I was progressed from patient care to team leading. During the time I was a team member I got to know the staff. I also got to know the floor and the equipment used. By the time I started team leading I felt fairly secure. I enjoyed my six-week orientation. I know I still have lots to learn but I'm comfortable and enjoy my work and co-workers.

Another wrote:

> It was a pleasure to come on duty. I knew exactly what I would be doing and how to do it. I found all employees and medical staff to be most helpful.

Following are other statements:

> For me, orientation was not that beneficial. I had worked here as a student. I received my team leadership here so I had rather just start working. If you can't just start working, then this is the best possible program.
>
> The most valuable part of the orientation program was the fact that it took place on the unit where I would work. I was actually working while learning and although the clinical nurse was there she did not hover over me.
>
> I did not think the program was complete in some respects. I had to be ward clerk for an hour one day and it was awful because I did not know what to do. I dreaded to graduate because I knew I would have to sit through a long orientation program watching pictures or listening to someone talk. It's just great, except for the desk.
>
> The only part I did not like was not knowing how to manage the desk when the unit secretary was away from the desk. Many times she went to lunch and there was no relief. When I had to substitute I felt frustrated. I think we should get training in managing the desk.
>
> I did not like the idea of being evaluated. I had just passed state boards and thought another evaluation was a waste of time. Actually I did not know when they were evaluating me, therefore it was not a painful experience, and I guess they have to know whether you can perform even if you do pass state boards. I found the experience very adequate.
>
> I believe my educational program prepared me very well for the activities I have been assigned to. I know I have much to learn but the staff is just wonderful, even the L.P.N.s and aides. They are all helpful.

Most of the evaluations were very positive. It may be argued that the nurse who does not admit needing orientation is the one who may need it most. The large number who expressed relief that they would not go through an inservice orientation is an indicator that most student nurses have a very negative attitude toward presently structured inservice.

CONCLUSION

It is recognized that this is a very small sample from which to draw a valid conclusion. When one considers the cost and marginal benefits of our present orientation programs, however, taking this risk would appear to be justified.

The satisfaction in the orientation program initiated, as evidenced by the evaluations, gives significant encouragement for experimentation.

Increasing independent responsibility for self-learning and freedom in performance must be accompanied by administrative encouragement and support.

As we place the responsibility for self-learning and competence on the individual, she will—in direct proportion—respond by self-learning and competence.

Economics

Change should never be motivated by economics alone, but programs that are an economic drain while providing marginal return for the investment in time and money do indicate need for further experimentation.

The program we had previously followed in orientation provided for the professional nurse from the Associate Degree Program or from the Diploma Program to receive four weeks of orientation by the inservice department. Two weeks of this time was spent in the inservice classroom. The remaining two weeks was spent on the hall, with the inservice instructor assisting and supervising the professional. The clinical nurse could not utilize the new employe in the work force in a meaningful way.

The baccalaureate graduate received a ten-week internship program. The first week was spent in the classroom. The second week was spent in working with and observing a team leader. So that a nurse clinician could spend her time with the internship program, we did not employ more than six to eight baccalaureate nurses at one time.

In calculating the cost of the former program in use, the following must be considered:

1. An inservice orientation director and two inservice instructors.
2. Two weeks of nonproductive man-hours per employee.
3. Eight weeks of no more than half time as productive man-hours.
4. The salary of a nurse clinician for ten weeks during an internship.

In contrast, the new program makes possible the following:

1. The new graduate can be a productive member of the nursing team after the first three days.
2. The inservice orientation section of the department of nursing service has been eliminated. This alone has resulted in a saving of more than thirty thousand dollars a year.
3. The hospital now has an orientation, training, and continuing education program. All hospital employees go through the three-day orientation program.
4. The department conducts other programs, which benefit all hospital employees.

References

Abdellah, Faye, Beland, Irene, Martin, Almeda, and Matheney, Ruth: Patient-centered approaches to nursing, New York, 1960, The Macmillan Publishers.

American Hospital Association: Functions of a hospital nursing service department, Chicago, 1962, American Hospital Association (unpaged folder).

American Nurses' Association: Inservice education for hospital nursing service personnel, New York, 1964, American Nurses' Association (unpaged folder).

American Nurses' Association: A position paper: educational preparation for nurse practitioners and assistants to nurses, New York, 1965, The Association.

Baker, Constance, and Kramer, Marlene: The exodus: can nursing afford it? The Journal of Nursing Administration, vol. I, no. 3, May, 1971. (This is focused mainly on those trained nurses who dropped out of nursing—50% left hospital nursing within two years; 28% withdrew from nursing practice altogether.)

Blumberg, Mark, and Dres, Jacqueline: Methods for assessing nursing care quality, Hospitals **37:**72-80, 1963.

Carter, Joan, Hilliard, Mildred, Castles, Mary, Stoll, Lee, and Cowan, Anne: Standards of nursing care: a guide for evaluation, New York, 1972, Springer Publishing Co., Inc.

Commission for Administrative Services in Hospitals (CASH): Staff utilization and control program orientation report, 1967.

Connor, Robert J.: A work sampling study of variations in nursing work load, Hospitals **35:**40-41, 111, May 1, 1961.

Dressler, Paul L.: College and university curriculum, Berkeley, Calif., 1971, McCutchan Publishing Corp.

Dunn, Michael D.: Nursing service study, Peoria, Ill., 1969, SDS Management Services.

Etzioni, Amitai, editor: The semi-professions and their organization; teachers, nurses, social workers, New York, 1969, Free Press.

Greenwood, E.: Attitudes of a profession, Social Work **2:**44, 1957.

Haimann, Theo.: Professional management, theory and practice, Boston, 1962, Houghton Mifflin Co.

Howland, Daniel, and McDowell, W. E.: The measurement of patient care: a conceptual framework, Nursing Research **13:**4-7, Winter, 1964.

Kellogg Foundation: SUM: an organizational approach to improved patient care, Battle Creek, Mich., 1971, The Foundation.

Kramer, Marlene: Collegiate graduate nurses in medical center hospitals: mutual challenge or duel, Nursing Research **18:**196-210, May-June, 1969.

Kramer, Marlene: Role conception and role deprivation of baccalaureate nurses and success in hospital nursing, Nursing Research **19:**428-439, Sept.-Oct., 1970.

Kramer, Marlene: Unpublished manuscript prepared for University of California, San Francisco Medical Center, 1972.

Kramer, Marlene: Reality shock: why nurses leave nursing, St. Louis, 1974, The C. V. Mosby Co.

Kramer, Samuel A.: The professions in the United States, Washington, D. C., 1955, U. S. Department of Health, Education and Welfare, Government Printing Office.

Kron, Thora: The management of patient care, Philadelphia, 1971, W. B. Saunders Co.

Lambertson, Eleanor: Graduate nurses' duty to define standards of good nursing care, Modern Hospital **1003:**130, July, 1964.

Lieberman, Myron: Education as a profession, Englewood Cliffs, N. J., 1956, Prentice-Hall, Inc.

Mayhew, Lewis B.: Graduate and professional

education, 1980. An essay written for the Carnegie Commission on Higher Education, New York, 1970, McGraw-Hill Book Co.

Murphy, Juanita: Theoretical issues in professional nursing, New York, 1971, Appleton-Century-Crofts, Educational Division, Meredith Corp.

National Commission for the Study of Nursing and Nursing Education: An abstract for action, New York, 1970, McGraw-Hill Book Co.

National League for Nursing: Inservice education for hospital nursing personnel, New York, 1958, National League for Nursing.

Palmer, Mary E.: Self-evaluation of nursing performance based on clinical practice objectives, Boston, 1962, Boston University Press.

Phaneuf, Maria: The nursing audit for evaluation of patient care, Nursing Outlook **14:** 51-54, June, 1966.

Schein, Edgar H.: Professional education: some new directions—Carnegie Commission on Higher Education, New York, 1972, McGraw-Hill Book Co.

U. S. Department of Health, Education and Welfare: Nurse Training Act of 1964. Program Review Report. Public Health Service Publication No. 1740, Washington, D. C., 1967, U. S. Government Printing Office.

U. S. Department of Health, Education and Welfare: Isolation techniques for use in hospitals, Atlanta, Ga., 1970, Center for Disease Control.

Wandelt, Mable A.: Quality patient care scale, Detroit, 1970, Wayne State University College of Nursing.

Index